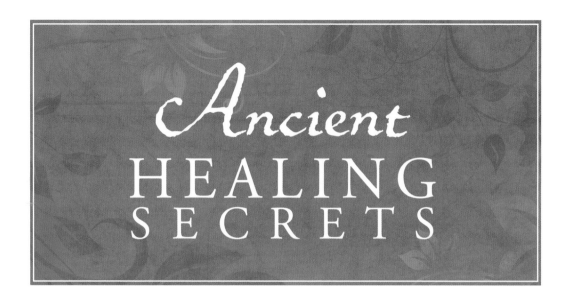

Ancient
HEALING
SECRETS

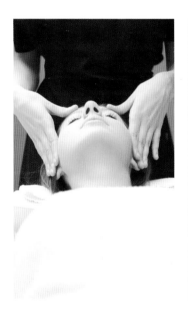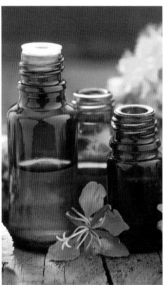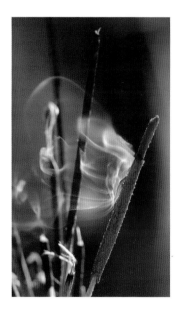

pil

Publications International, Ltd.

Cover and interior art: Shutterstock.com

Contributing writers: Gayle Alleman, M.S., R.D.; Janice Deal; Kathi Keville; Jeffrey Laign; Dianne Molvig; Bill Schoenbart, L.Ac.; Jill Stansbury, N.D.

Louis Weber, CEO
Publications International, Ltd.
7373 North Cicero Avenue
Lincolnwood, Illinois 60712

Permission is never granted for commercial purposes.

ISBN: 978-1-68022-192-3

Manufactured in China.

8 7 6 5 4 3 2 1

Note: This publication is only intended to provide general information. The information is specifically not intended to be substitute for medical diagnosis or treatment by your physician or other healthcare professional. You should always consult your own physician or other healthcare professionals about any medical questions, diagnosis, or treatment. (Products vary among manufacturers. Please check labels carefully to confirm that the products you use are appropriate for your condition.)

The information obtained by you from this publication should not be relied upon for any personal, nutritional, or medical decision. You should consult an appropriate professional for specific advice tailored to your specific situation. PIL makes no representation or warranties, express or implied, with respect to your use of this information.

In no event shall PIL or its affiliates or advertisers be liable for any direct, indirect, punitive, incidental, special, or consequential damages, or any damages whatsoever including, without limitation, damages for personal injury, death, damage to property or loss of profits, arising out of or in any way connected with the use of any of the above-referenced information or otherwise arising out of use of this publication.

CONTENTS

INTRODUCTION 4

TRADITIONAL CHINESE MEDICINE 6

MASSAGE 45

CHIROPRACTIC 53

REFLEXOLOGY 59

COLD AND HEAT TREATMENTS 69

EXERCISE 77

TRADITIONS FROM INDIA:
AYURVEDIC MEDICINE AND YOGA 85

HERBS FOR HEALTH AND HEALING 93

AROMATHERAPY 123

KITCHEN CURE-ALLS 153

COMMON CONDITIONS 167

In Spring 2015, a 1,000-year old herbal remedy that combined garlic, onion, wine, and bile from a cow's stomach made the news in a big way. Researchers tested this ancient English remedy for eye infections against the modern superbug MRSA. The results were amazing—the remedy was highly effective. The incident raised an intriguing question: as bacteria become resistant to modern antibiotics, can solutions be found not only in modern laboratories but in the distant past? On a more general level, if we broaden our understanding of what medicine entails, might we find additional treatments for stubborn problems?

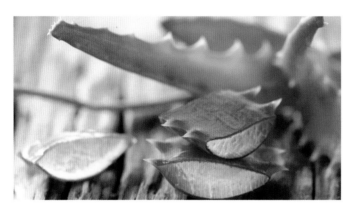 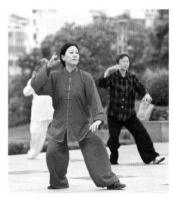

Humans have been working to combat infections, cure diseases, and treat injuries for thousands of years, often through trial and error. Not everything from the past worked—sometimes, "lost" knowledge was lost for a reason. In many cases we've learned more than we once knew about how to treat a particular disease. However, in other cases, the ancient remedies still prove astoundingly effective—and they can be less costly and come with fewer side effects than modern Western medications. In this book, we look at some of the medical knowledge that's been passed down through the centuries to determine what can still be applied today.

In two chapters, one on Traditional Chinese Medicine and another on the Ayurvedic tradition from India, you'll find an overview on these comprehensive medical systems that have developed over centuries and are still in use today. Other chapters, such as Massage, Exercise, and Cold and Heat Treatments, look at some basic healing ideas that have been used through many cultures over time. The chapters Herbs, Aromatherapy, and "Kitchen Cure-Alls" (garlic, vinegar, honey, and olive oil), will provide you with both historical information and ideas and recipes for how you can make your own household remedies. The final section of the book, Common Conditions, will give you a selection of time-tested remedies from around the world that you might use to address common problems such as headaches, colds, and stomach aches. (Note that, if you have chronic health problems or are taking other medications or supplements, you'll want to discuss any potential remedies with your health care practitioner first. Some herbal remedies, for example, are contraindicated for people who take certain medications.)

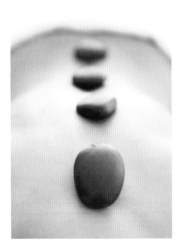 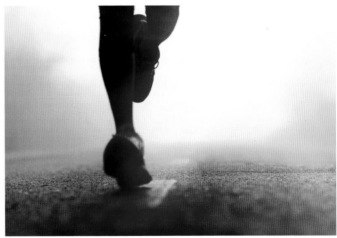

Whether you're looking for information about the theories behind acupuncture and moxibustion (page 26), trying to determine what kind of massage is right for you (page 45), or finding ways to alleviate the symptoms of the common cold (page 169), this book will act as your guide. Along the way, you will find both fascinating historical tidbits and practical advice. Just turn the page to begin uncovering knowledge that will intrigue you and inform you—and that might just change your life.

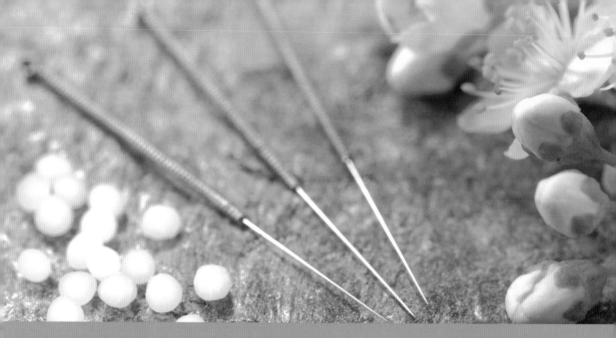

TRADITIONAL CHINESE MEDICINE

Archeological excavations reveal that human beings lived in China more than a million years ago. These primitive people spent most of their time on basic survival: hunting, locating and preparing plants for food, building shelters, and defending themselves. It's easy to imagine that over time, they'd have sampled most of the local plants in their search for food. In time, an oral record evolved that identified those plants that made good food, those that were useful for building, those that had an effect on illness, and those that were poisonous. Through trial and error, a primitive form of herbal medicine and dietary therapy was taking shape in China.

Fire also played a central role in their lives as a source of warmth, fuel, and light. As our ancestors huddled around fires, it was only natural that they would discover the healing powers of heat. Those powers would have been especially evident for ailments such as arthritis, for which heat provides immediate relief. This was the origin of the art of moxibustion, the therapeutic application of heat to treat a wide variety of conditions.

These ancient people must have experienced a variety of injuries during their rugged lives. A natural reaction to pain is to rub or press on the affected area. This hands-on therapy gradually evolved into a system of therapeutic manipulation. People discovered that pressing on certain points on the body had wide-ranging effects. When they began to use pieces of sharpened bone or stone to enhance the sensation, acupuncture was born.

WRITTEN HISTORY

The development of a written record of Chinese medicine has evolved mostly over the last 3,000 years. Archeological digs from the Shang Dynasty (1,000 B.C.) have revealed medical writings inscribed on divination bones: Early shamans, mostly women, used scapula bones to perform divination rites; later these bones were also used for writing. The discovery in 1973 of 11 medical texts written on silk has shed some light on the sophisticated practices of that early period of Chinese history. Dated to 168 B.C., the texts discuss diet, exercise, moxibustion, and herbal therapy. Liberally mixed with shamanistic magic, an extensive text, *Prescriptions for Fifty-two Ailments*, describes the pharmacologic effects of herbs and foods.

Also dating from about this time is the legend of Shen Nong, the Emperor of Agriculture, who tasted 100 herbs daily to assess their qualities. (He is said to have been poisoned many times in the course of his investigations.) The book that is attributed to him is known as the *Classic of the Agriculture Emperor's Materia Medica*. It lists 365 medicines, comprising 252 plants, 67 animals, and 46 minerals. Tao Hong-Jing, the editor of the version of Shen Nong's materia medica in use today, divided the herbs into three classes. The upper-class herbs are nontoxic tonics that strengthen and nourish the body, the middle-grade herbs are tonics with therapeutic qualities, and the lower grade consists of herbs that treat disease or possess some toxicity. This classification system gives a glimpse into an important principle in traditional Chinese medicine: It is better to strengthen the body and prevent disease than to fight illness once it has already taken hold. Ignoring preventive health care and waiting to treat disease was considered as foolish as waiting until you are thirsty to dig a well.

By A.D. 400, the basic foundations of traditional Chinese medicine had been put into written form. The most important book compiled between 300 B.C. and A.D. 400 is *The Yellow Emperor's Inner Classic (Huang Di Nei Jing)*. The work is divided into two books: *Simple Questions* and *Spiritual Axis*. The first book deals with general theoretical principles, while the second more specifically describes the principles of acupuncture and the treatment of disease. Remarkably, this ancient work is still valid; it forms the foundation for the contemporary practice of traditional Chinese medicine. For example, the Nei Jing states that cold diseases should be treated with hot herbs, and hot diseases should be treated with cold herbs. This principle is still followed today in clinical practice.

By the second century A.D., physicians all over China were compiling writings of the latest discoveries in acupuncture and herbal medicine. It was during this time that the famous physician Hua Tuo wrote about his unique system of acupuncture points, which is still in use. He was also a pioneer in recommending exercise as a method of maintaining wellness. He is quoted as saying "a running stream never goes bad," meaning exercise moves qi and prevents the stagnation that leads to disease.

Another pioneer of the time was Zhang Zhongjing, who wrote *Treatise on Febrile and Miscellaneous Diseases* after witnessing an epidemic that ravaged his city. This highly regarded physician developed a system of diagnosis so sophisticated that it is used by practitioners in modern hospitals 1,700 years after his death.

PROGRESS OF MEDICINE IN CHINA

Between the 2nd and 5th centuries A.D., China experienced a period marked by war and political turmoil. One of the ironies of war is that it has a tendency to lead to advances in medicine. The periodic times of unrest in Chinese history were no exception, as the increased need for practical, convenient, effective remedies led to further developments in medical treatment. During the time of the Tang Dynasty (618–907 A.D.), China's Imperial Medical Bureau established departments of Acupuncture, Pharmacology, and Medical Specialties, and numerous additional treatises and compilations of medical knowledge and experience were prepared.

In the Five Dynasties period (907–1368 A.D.), advancements in printing techniques led to a dramatic increase in the publication of medical texts. One of the important books of the period was *Canon on the Origin of Acupuncture and Moxibustion,* in which Wang Zhizhong incorporated the clinical experiences of the practitioners of folk medicine. During the Ming Dynasty (1368–1644), many medical specialists compiled the works of their forebears, further expanding the extensive base of medical knowledge. The most famous physician of the period was Li Shi Zheng (1518–1593). His most incredible achievement was his 40-year effort in writing the *Ben Cao Gong Mu (General Catalog of Herbs),* a monumental work published after his death. Consisting of 52 volumes at the time of its printing, the *Ben Cao Gong Mu* remains an important reference for traditional Chinese herbalists.

The integration of new techniques with ancient understanding continued until the 19th century, when Western colonial powers derided traditional medicine as primitive and outdated. The Communist party came to power in the mid-20th century, bringing much turmoil to China; however, the Communists saw the need to promote traditional Chinese medicine to avoid dependence on the West. A great need for traditional doctors arose since there were far too few Western-trained physicians to serve the huge population: only 10,000 Western-trained doctors were available to serve 400 million people. Traditional Chinese medicine began a course of revival that continues today.

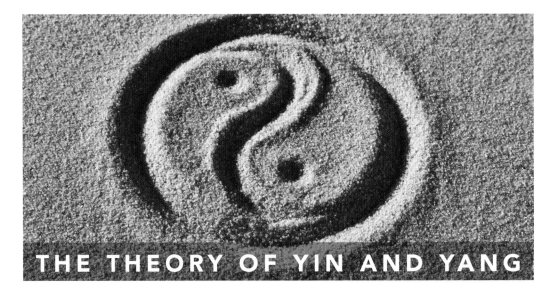

THE THEORY OF YIN AND YANG

Through patient observation of the forces of nature, the Taoists who developed the system of traditional Chinese medicine saw the universe as a unified field, constantly moving and changing while maintaining its oneness. This constant state of change was explained through the theory of yin and yang. According to the theory, nature expresses itself in an endless cycle of polar opposites such as day and night, moisture and dryness, heat and cold, and activity and rest. Yin phenomena are those that exhibit the nurturing qualities of darkness, rest, moisture, cold, and structure. Yang phenomena have qualities of energy such as light, activity, dryness, heat, and function. Everything in nature exhibits varying combinations of both yin and yang. For example, the morning fog (yin) is dissipated by the heat of the sun (yang). Any phenomenon within nature can be understood in relation to another; one will always be yin or yang in comparison with the other.

Some of the basic principles of yin and yang:

- **Everything in nature can be expressed as the opposition of yin and yang.** This is the energizing force of all aspects of nature. It is dynamic and the basic foundation for change in nature. Yin and yang are also relative terms: A forest fire is more yang than a campfire; a campfire is more yang than a spark. Nothing is purely yin or yang; it is always a matter of comparison.

- **Yin and yang are interdependent.** Even though yin and yang are opposites, one has no meaning without the other. For example, day would have no meaning without night; heat cannot be understood without knowing what cold feels like; fever and chills can't be determined without experiencing the normal body temperature.

- **Yin creates yang; yang creates yin.** Numerous examples of this principle can be seen in nature. For example, on a hot summer day (yang), there is a sudden thunderstorm (yin). A person may get symptoms of chills and a runny nose (yin) that turn into a fever with a sore throat (yang).

- **Yin and yang mutually control each other.** This is the basic mechanism of balance in nature and the human body. When the body gets overheated from exercise, the pores open and sweating lowers the temperature. When the body gets too cold due to exposure, the muscles shiver to generate heat.

Since the Taoists believe that everything is part of the oneness of the universe, they make no distinction between the external forces of nature and the internal processes of the human body, believing that "the macrocosm exists within the microcosm." In other words, any process or change that can be witnessed in nature can also be seen in the body.

For example, a person who eats cold food (yin) on a cold, damp day (yin) may experience excessive mucus (yin). Similarly, a person who performs strenuous activity (yang) on a hot day (yang) might experience dehydration with a fever (yang). Some of the traditional diagnoses sound like weather reports, such as "wind and cold with dampness" (a yin condition) or a "deficiency of moisture leading to fire" (a yang pattern). These diagnostic descriptions illustrate the principle that the body experiences the same fluctuations of yin and yang as the environment.

The internal organs also have their own balance of yin and yang. Yin functions tend to be nourishing, cooling, building, and relaxing and relate to the structure, or substance, of the organs. Yang qualities tend to be energizing, warming, consuming, and stimulating and relate to the functional activity of the organs. For example, the kidneys are considered the source of yin (water) and yang (fire, or metabolism) for the entire body. If the kidney yin is deficient or depleted, a person can experience hot flashes and night sweats, as occurs in menopause when estrogen (yin) levels decline. This is due to insufficient moisture (yin) to keep the metabolic fire (yang), which keeps the body warm, under control. Think of running a car engine with insufficient oil; the engine will overheat due to a deficiency of this yin-like lubricant. A deficiency of kidney yang produces such symptoms as cold hands and feet and a general lack of vitality. These symptoms, which often occur with age, are due to insufficient metabolic fire (yang) to infuse the entire body with energy and warmth, dispersing cold and fatigue (yin).

Traditional Chinese medicine applies this ancient theory of yin and yang in clinical practice. Since all the organs have similar yin and yang aspects, it is possible to monitor and adjust the yin and yang levels of all parts of the body, maintaining a high level of vitality and preventing disease. This is achieved not only with herbs but with changes in diet and lifestyle. In this way, the ancient observations of the Taoists have practical applications in our own quest for wellness.

THE VITAL SUBSTANCES

In traditional Chinese medicine, the body and mind are inseparable. Composed of a number of vital substances—qi (pronounced chee), blood, essence, and body fluids—the body and mind express their qualities through the functions of the internal organs. Ranging from tangible, visible substances to subtle, intangible forces, these basic elements of the body/mind are responsible for all aspects of human life—physical, mental, emotional, and spiritual. Their intimate involvement in human activity makes them an essential part of physiology, and recognition and understanding of them are an essential part of diagnosis.

QI

Although qi plays a central role in traditional Chinese medicine, it is extremely difficult to define. It is best to understand it in terms of its functions and activities, where it is more readily perceived. Situated somewhere between matter and energy, qi has the qualities of both. It has substance without structure, and it possesses energy qualities but can't be measured. It is the fundamental power underlying all the activities of nature as well as the vital life force of the human body. For example, the force of a thunderstorm can be understood in terms of its qi: The power of qi can be observed in the fallen trees and buildings in the storm's aftermath. Similarly, the strength of the digestive organs can be determined in relation to their qi by evaluating the appetite, color of the tongue, strength of the pulse, and the body's response to nutrition.

The flow of qi through the body occurs within a closed system of channels, or meridians. There are twelve major meridians, and they correspond to the twelve organ systems: six yin organs and six yang organs. Traditional organ theory pairs yin and yang organs according to their structure and function and the interconnection of their meridians.

THE FLOW OF QI

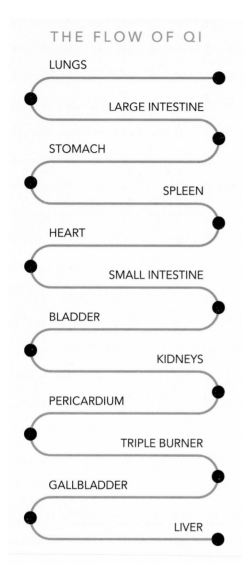

LUNGS

LARGE INTESTINE

STOMACH

SPLEEN

HEART

SMALL INTESTINE

BLADDER

KIDNEYS

PERICARDIUM

TRIPLE BURNER

GALLBLADDER

LIVER

In addition, eight extra meridians are interconnected with all the channels. This network of meridians allows the qi, or life force, to reach all the tissues and organs, providing nourishment, warmth, and energy to all parts of the body. The flow of qi travels from channel to channel, passing through all the meridians every 24 hours. Although the meridians are deep within the body, points along them are accessible from the surface of the skin. It is the manipulation of these points by means of pressure, heat, or needles that is the basis for acupressure, moxibustion, and acupuncture, respectively. The qi that flows through the meridians can be manipulated at the acupuncture points, bringing healing energy to organs that need it and moving energy away from areas that are impaired due to stagnation of qi.

TYPES OF QI

Chinese medicine traditionally divides qi into various types, depending on its source and function. The original source of this life force is a person's parents, and the qi inherited from them is known as prenatal qi. Prenatal qi, the basic constitution of a human being, depends on genetics and the quality of the parents' lives at the time of conception and during pregnancy. This qi is the person's heritage, and it cannot be replenished; however, healthy lifestyle, diet, and breathing practices can conserve prenatal qi and slow down its depletion.

Postnatal qi, or acquired qi, is derived from the digestion of food and extracted from the air we breathe. Combined with prenatal qi, it forms the totality of the body's power to perform all the vital processes of life. One of the functions of the lungs is to extract qi from air and incorporate it into the storehouse of postnatal qi. The strength of postnatal qi depends on a number of factors: the strength of lung qi, the quality of the air, and the performance of breathing exercises such as qi gong, which enhances the lungs' ability to extract qi from air. When lung qi is deficient, a person can experience symptoms of fatigue, shortness of breath, pallor, and frequent colds. The other factor in building strong postnatal qi is the quality of the food we eat and the strength of our digestive organs, especially the spleen. When spleen qi is weak, symptoms of fatigue, lack of appetite, sluggishness, and loose stools can occur. When the diet lacks essential nutrients and variety, the extraction of qi is impaired even if spleen qi is strong.

When both spleen qi and lung qi are strong, and the quality of our air and food are high, postnatal qi can grow. Herbs that tonify lung and spleen qi, along with breathing practices such as qi gong, further increase the accumulation of postnatal qi. In this way, even a person with a weak inherited constitution (prenatal qi) can experience a life of health and vitality.

The totality of qi that results from the combination of prenatal and postnatal qi is known as true qi. Responsible for all the functions of the body, true qi takes different forms. From the clinical perspective, two of these forms of qi are especially significant: nutritive qi and protective qi.

Nutritive qi circulates in the meridians and nourishes the organs. Acupuncture manipulates this qi to affect organ function. Specific points along the meridians are needled, pressed, or warmed (by means of moxibustion) to achieve specific effects in the organs. For example, a point below the knee is manipulated traditionally to treat appendicitis, often eliminating the symptoms when the condition is caught before infection sets in. When a Chinese surgeon performing appendectomies needled this point on his patients, he found that the intestines contracted rhythmically on either side of the appendix.

The other important subdivision of true qi is protective qi, or wei qi. Believed to flow between the skin and muscles, wei qi is responsible for defending the body from external pathogens that attack the body. Although first described thousands of years ago, wei qi accurately describes the body's immune system. Herbs traditionally used to tonify wei qi have a powerful effect in strengthening the body's resistance to disease and increasing immune function. Certain acupuncture points have similar effects on immune function.

DISORDERS OF QI

Chinese medicine seeks to ensure that the levels, direction, and flow of qi are all appropriate for their particular organs. The various disorders of qi that can occur involve deficiency, sinking, stagnation, or incorrect movement of qi. The symptoms of qi deficiency are common to all the types of qi disorders: fatigue, pallor, and lethargy. When the qi of an organ is deficient, the specific functions of that organ are also impaired. For example, the spleen is responsible for appetite and digestion; spleen qi deficiency produces poor appetite and loose stools. Lung qi is responsible for the strength of respiration; when it is deficient, a person experiences shortness of breath and a chronic cough. Treatment focuses on strengthening, or tonifying, the qi of the affected organs.

In disorders of sinking qi, the qi that holds organs in place has insufficient strength to do its job. The result is sagging, prolapsed organs, such as the uterus, transverse colon, or rectum. Specific acupuncture points and herbs can correct this type of imbalance.

When qi is stagnant, the functions of an organ are impaired due to a blockage in its qi flow. The liver is the organ most often affected by qi stagnation. Since the liver is in charge of the smooth flow of emotion, stagnant liver qi frequently results in irritability and anger. Because there is sufficient qi, tonifying in these cases would make the situation worse, so treatment focuses on moving qi away from the area.

In rebellious qi, the normal direction of organ qi is reversed. Each organ has a normal direction of qi flow; for example, the lungs and stomach move qi downward, while the spleen moves qi upward. Rebellious lung qi results in coughing or wheezing; rebellious stomach qi produces symptoms of nausea, belching, or vomiting; and rebellious spleen qi produces diarrhea.

BLOOD

In traditional Chinese medicine, blood has some parallels to its Western counterpart, such as its function of circulating through the body and nourishing the organs. However, it also has some very subtle functions in traditional Chinese medicine, such as providing a substantial foundation for the mind and improving sensitivity of the sensory organs. In other words, a deficiency of blood causes an impairment in mental function, leading to poor memory, anxiety, and insomnia. Blood deficiency can also impair the senses, especially the eyes, causing blurry vision.

When blood is deficient, symptoms such as dry skin and hair, inflexible tendons, and various emotional and reproductive imbalances can occur, depending on the organs involved. Since qi and blood are so closely related, a deficiency or stagnation of one of the substances often leads to the same type of imbalance in the other one.

BLOOD AND QI

Closely aligned with qi, blood has a complementary relationship with it. The saying, "Blood is the mother of qi, and qi is the leader of blood," refers to the fact that without blood, qi has no fundamental nutritional basis; without qi, the body cannot form or circulate blood, and the blood would fail to stay within the vessels. The two are considered to flow together through the body.

BODY FLUIDS

Body fluids refer to all the fluids in the body, such as sweat, tears, saliva, and various secretions and lubricants. The spleen and stomach regulate the formation of fluids, which are considered byproducts of digestion, while the intestines and bladder are involved in their excretion. The lungs regulate body fluids from above, and the kidneys are in charge of their metabolism throughout the body. Fluids consist of two basic types: clear thin fluids known as jin, and thick viscous fluids known as ye. Jin is distributed mostly to the muscles and skin, keeping them moist and nourished. Ye acts as a lubricant to the joints and nourishes the brain. Jin ye is the collective term for all the body fluids.

Because of the relationship between the organs and body fluids, a traditional Chinese medicine practitioner can extrapolate a wealth of information about organ function from the condition of the jin ye. For this reason, the initial interview includes questions about thirst, urination, color of fluids, and the amount and timing of sweating.

The body fluids also have an intimate relationship with qi. Since qi is involved in the transformation of fluids, deficient qi can lead to fluid retention or excessive sweating. Conversely, fluid stagnation can impair qi circulation, and profuse loss of body fluid can lead to a severe deficiency of qi. For this reason, herbs that induce sweating are used cautiously in people who are qi deficient.

ESSENCE AND SPIRIT (JING AND SHEN)

Stored in the kidneys, essence (jing) is the subtle substance that is responsible for growth, development, and reproduction. Prenatal essence is inherited from the parents, and it is the original substance of life. It cannot be increased, but it can be conserved through a healthy lifestyle and moderation. It can be supplemented with postnatal essence, which is derived from nutrition. When the essence is strong, a child grows and develops normally and enjoys healthy brain function and strong immunity and fertility as an adult.

Spirit (shen) is a person's innate vitality. It can be considered the soul, but it also has a material aspect. When an individual has healthy shen, the eyes have the glow of life and the mind is clear. Since the heart is the resting place for the spirit, disturbances in shen are typically diagnosed as heart imbalances. A mild shen syndrome appears with a heart blood deficiency, with signs of forgetfulness, insomnia, fatigue, and restlessness. In a more serious shen syndrome, "heat phlegm confusing the heart," the individual may be violent, with red face and eyes; the Western diagnosis of this condition might be psychosis.

THE INTERNAL ORGANS

The internal organs are responsible for the vital functions of the human body. The understanding and description of the internal organ structures and systems in traditional Chinese medicine is remarkably sophisticated, considering the fact that traditional organ theory was developed during Confucian times (approximately 559–479 B.C.). In this period, it was considered a violation of the sanctity of life to perform dissections, so the entire organ theory was developed on the basis of how the body functions. The body was viewed in a holistic sense, with the understanding that all functions necessary to maintain health were innately present within its internal organs. By means of careful observation, the Taoists were able to perceive functional relationships among seemingly unrelated activities, actions, emotions, and sensory perceptions.

The function and structure of the vital organs in traditional Chinese medicine differ from that of similarly named organs in Western medicine. It's true that in some cases, the functional relationships closely parallel those established in Western medicine. For example, the Taoists reasoned that "the kidneys govern water." Both traditional Chinese and Western medical systems recognize that the kidneys play an essential role in filtering and expelling waste water through the urinary bladder. But Chinese medical theory discusses the organs based not only on their function but on their relationship with other organs. In traditional organ theory, the kidneys are also responsible for reproduction and fertility; this theory has no counterpart in the Western anatomic concept of the organ. Yet, herbs that nourish "kidney essence" are quite effective clinically in promoting fertility. It is important to let each medical system stand on its own rather than attempting to create a one-to-one correspondence between Western anatomy and the Taoist functional organ systems.

In traditional Chinese medicine, the five yin organs, or solid (zang) organs, are the lungs, spleen, heart, liver, and kidneys. The pericardium is sometimes considered a sixth yin organ. The yin organs produce, transform, and store qi, blood, body fluids, and essence.

The six yang organs, or hollow (fu) organs, are generally considered to be less significant in their functions than are the yin organs. The yang organs serve primarily to separate impure substances from food and then drain them out of the body as waste material. Each yang organ is paired with a yin organ. For example, the spleen and the stomach together encompass the digestive process. The stomach performs the yang function of processing the food and passing it on; the spleen performs the yin function of extracting nourishment from the food and transforming it into qi and blood.

The "extra" or "curious" organs are so named because their existence can be confirmed through observation, but they don't fall into any particular category. They are the marrow, bones, blood vessels, brain, uterus, and gallbladder. Although the gallbladder is classified as a yang organ, it is also considered a curious organ since it is the only yang organ that stores a vital substance (bile). The marrow is a vital essence stored by the kidneys. It is related to growth and development and nourishes the brain. The functions of the other organs parallel their Western counterparts.

PATTERNS OF DISHARMONY

Over the centuries, a sophisticated system of diagnosis has evolved in traditional Chinese medicine. By following various established diagnostic procedures, a practitioner of traditional Chinese medicine can construct a detailed picture of the status of all the internal organs. To identify a pattern of disharmony, the physician will assess the status of the organs, gradually uncovering the cause of the disease by grouping the symptoms into traditional patterns.

During the initial patient visit, the practitioner must organize all of the seemingly unrelated facts gathered about a patient's condition, gradually refining this information into diagnostic categories. At first, the practitioner organizes the evidence loosely into general categories known as the eight parameters, which consist of four groups of polarities: yin and yang, heat and cold, internal and external, excess and deficiency. This eight-parameter diagnosis is the basic foundation for all diagnostic categories. It gives the practitioner a general overview of the patient's disease, or a pattern of disharmony. Once the practitioner has grouped the symptoms according to the eight parameters, he or she can further refine the diagnosis to determine the condition of the vital substances and the internal organs. In this way, the diagnosis evolves from a general image into a specific, clear description of the individual patient's physiologic processes.

THE CAUSES OF DISHARMONY

Practitioners of traditional Chinese medicine consider a number of factors in determining the cause of illness. Some of these causes are considered external, as in the six pernicious influences: wind, cold, heat, dryness, dampness and summer heat. Other causes are considered internal, as in the seven emotions: anger, joy, worry, pensiveness, sadness, fear, and shock. Other factors that play a role in the development of disease are diet, lifestyle, and accidents.

Once a practitioner establishes a general diagnosis, taking into account the eight parameters, the vital substances, and the pernicious influences, the next step is to determine which organ systems are affected. This logical procedure leads to a final diagnosis that is specific enough to enable the physician to prepare a focused treatment plan. For example, a patient may have chronic night sweats, irritability, and thirst—general signs of yin deficiency—but the practitioner still does not know which organ system to nourish at this point. Keeping in mind the normal functions of the organs, the practitioner might find further symptoms of palpitations, insomnia, and poor memory, concluding that the yin deficiency affects mostly the heart. The treatment plan would then include an herbal formula to nourish heart yin.

CASE STUDY

Joe is a 40-year-old executive with a high-stress lifestyle, often working overtime. He drinks coffee frequently to "keep up his energy," and his meals often consist of pastries from a vending machine. His colleagues complain he is prone to bouts of sudden anger for no good reason, so they keep their distance. He always seems to have a stiff neck, and his face and eyes are often red. His doctor is very concerned about his high blood pressure, and his wife has warned him that she will leave him if he doesn't stop yelling at her at the slightest provocation.

This is a classic case of excess liver yang or fire, caused by Joe's lifestyle and diet. The symptoms can be alleviated with acupuncture and herbal therapy. However, to achieve lasting healing, Joe's life needs a major overhaul. In addition to working less, the most important change he must make is to eliminate coffee, since it directly overheats the liver. Since caffeine withdrawal can also cause similar symptoms, green tea is a good substitute at first. Although it still has some caffeine, green tea has a cooling energy that disturbs the liver far less. And it can be decreased or eliminated later without causing discomfort.

A well-balanced diet is also essential, since a deficient diet harms the liver and also leads to qi deficiency and a consequent craving for stimulants. Exercise and stress-reduction techniques will also help lower blood pressure and create an appetite for good food. Once Joe's liver cools down with lifestyle changes, acupuncture, and herbal therapy, he will be much less prone to outbursts of anger. He can then take cooling tonics such as American ginseng, which will give him extra energy without creating all the side effects of coffee.

DIAGNOSIS IN TRADITIONAL CHINESE MEDICINE

It is important to remember that the functions of organs in traditional Chinese medicine may overlap those of their Western counterparts, but they also have totally unrelated functions. For this reason, it is dangerous to attempt to find a standard correspondence between the two. For example, a chest cold might be diagnosed as a lung condition under both systems, but asthma might be a kidney condition in traditional Chinese medical diagnostics. Both medical systems stand on their own strengths, but an attempt to artificially link the two can often make them less effective. Attempting to treat the flu simply with Chinese herbs that have antiviral qualities is less effective than getting an accurate diagnosis—wind heat, for example—and using a traditional formula for that wind heat.

Diagnosis in traditional Chinese medicine may appear to be simply a grouping of symptoms, but the elegance of Chinese medicine is that a diagnosis automatically indicates a treatment strategy. For example, a woman experiencing menopause may have hot flashes, night sweats, thirst, and irritability; this group of symptoms leads to a diagnosis of kidney yin deficiency with heat. This diagnosis immediately points to the indicated therapy: Tonify kidney yin and clear deficiency heat. Since standard formulas are available for this pattern, an accurate diagnosis enables a practitioner to prescribe a treatment that has been proved safe and effective for thousands of years.

A practitioner can obtain all of the information needed to diagnose disease through inquiry and external observation. The four basic categories of diagnostic observation are looking, listening and smelling, asking, and touching. Simply by employing these four areas of investigation, traditional practitioners can accurately assess physical and emotional imbalances of the internal organs and reestablish harmony. It is important to remember that diagnostic indicators are always viewed holistically—that is, in total and in relation to the whole person. For example, fatigue is a symptom of qi or blood deficiency, but fatigue is also a symptom in a case of wind cold. If a person with wind cold was mistakenly diagnosed with qi deficiency, he might be given ginseng, a strong tonic that would make the symptoms much worse. A careful practitioner would note that the person's pulse was strong and floating, a sign of wind cold, while a person with qi deficiency would have a deep and weak pulse. While it is necessary to learn the individual diagnostic patterns, it is crucial to remember that any sign or symptom must be viewed in relation to the whole person.

Looking: Practitioners look at the face, inspecting the quality of the spirit (shen) that can be seen in the eyes. Changes in facial skin color can also provide the practitioner with clues. Practitioners look at the body as well, as the overall physique of the patient may provide clues. The lips and the tongue can also provide vital diagnostic information.

Listening and smelling: The practitioner listens to the patient's speech, their breathing, and other bodily sounds such as gastrointestinal signs. Odors of the breath, urine, stools, vomit, and sweat can also provide clues.

Asking: This is an exceptionally important part of diagnosis. The practitioner must listen to the patient and get an accurate picture of the patient's past medical history, their lifestyle, and their current complaint.

Touching: The art of touch in traditional Chinese medicine is highly sophisticated and includes the palpation of areas of pain and diagnostic points and the reading of the patient's pulse.

TREATMENTS IN TRADITIONAL CHINESE MEDICINE

Once practitioners of traditional Chinese medicine make a diagnosis, they have the following options available to treat their patients: acupuncture, herbal medicine, moxibustion, cupping, exercise therapy, massage techniques, and dietary therapy. The most common therapeutic modalities are acupuncture and herbal medicine, which have such a wide range of applications, they are appropriate for most conditions. Moxibustion (the application of heat to acupuncture points or injured areas) is also widely used, while cupping (the application of suction cups to remove stagnation from an area) is often employed as an adjunct therapy for pain and stagnation. A traditional massage technique known as tui na has a profound effect on the musculoskeletal system. Sophisticated forms of exercise, or movement, therapy known as qi gong and tai qi, can be used to direct healing qi to specific areas of the body. Finally, dietary therapy is an important aspect of all healing systems, and Chinese medicine is no exception. Foods are grouped according to the organ systems they affect and whether they are hot or cold, damp or dry, yin or yang. Practitioners often advise patients about which foods to eat and which to avoid for their particular imbalance.

ACUPUNCTURE

The practice of acupuncture is based on the flow of qi, or vital energy, through pathways in the body known as channels, or meridians. Twelve regular meridians correspond to each of the six yin and six yang organs—the spleen meridian to the spleen organ, the large intestine meridian to the large intestine organ, and so on. Eight extra meridians are also used in acupuncture therapy. Disharmony in an organ often shows up in its corresponding meridian: A person experiencing a heart

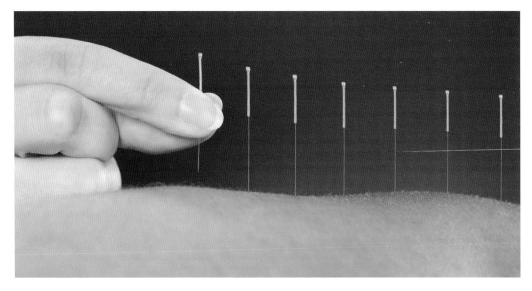

attack may also have a sensation of pain and numbness that travels down the arm into the little finger, closely following the path of the heart meridian. Practitioners palpate a diagnostic point on the corresponding meridian to assess the health of its related organ. In other cases, the meridians themselves are treated. A practitioner might treat a sore shoulder by increasing the flow of qi and blood through the large intestine, lung, and triple burner meridians. The organs related to these meridians may be completely healthy; these meridians are selected because they pass through the injured shoulder area.

Although they flow deep within the body, each meridian has specific points that can be accessed from the surface of the body. There are 361 such acupuncture points on the meridians, as well as numerous "extraordinary" points that may or may not be located on a regular channel. Acupuncture points can be stimulated by means of pressure, heat, or needling. Each point has a specific set of functions. Some of these functions have local effects, while some are systemic (affecting the body's systems as a whole). For example, the stomach meridian consists of 45 points, stretching from the head to the toes. A point just below the knee known as Dubi, or Stomach 35, is used almost exclusively for knee pain (a local effect), while the point just three inches below it, known as Zusanli (Stomach 36), has a systemic function. One of the most important points in acupuncture, Zusanli is used to treat stomach pain, vomiting, indigestion, diarrhea, constipation, dizziness, fatigue, and low immunity. Needling it often relieves stomach pain immediately.

Acupuncture has been practiced since ancient times with needles made from stone, wood, ivory, or bone. Modern practitioners use surgical-quality stainless steel needles with a handle wound with wire for a better grip. Some needles are plated with silver, gold, or copper to achieve special effects from the treatment, such as tonification or sedation, but the majority of needles are pure steel. In the past, needles were placed in an autoclave, a device used to sterilize dental and surgical tools, after each use. However, with the increase in prevalence of hepatitis and AIDS/HIV, most practitioners in the West now use presterilized disposable needles to ensure absolute safety. The needles are used only once and then discarded as medical waste, which gives peace of mind to the patients, practitioners, and insurance companies.

Acupuncture is used to treat a number of conditions, but it is especially well known for its treatment of pain; it is so effective for pain relief, it is even used as a substitute for anesthesia in some surgical procedures in Chinese hospitals!

THE TECHNIQUE

Many people are surprised to learn that acupuncture is relatively painless. Unlike hypodermic needles, which are hollow and much larger, acupuncture needles can be as fine as a human hair. Many times, a patient is not even aware a needle has been inserted, especially when it is placed in areas with relatively few sensory nerves, such as the back. In a typical acupuncture treatment, the patient lies down, and the practitioner inserts needles in points that have the desired effect on the body. The patient senses heaviness, movement, or an "electrical" impulse that signals the "arrival of qi." After a few minutes, the patient typically feels a sense of calmness and well-being; many people fall asleep.

After a period of 20 minutes to an hour, the practitioner removes the needles and advises the patient to avoid strenuous activity for a few hours to let the treatment settle in. Depending on the individual and the condition, one treatment might be sufficient, or the patient may need to return a number of times. Results can range from mild improvement to seemingly miraculous recovery. In almost all cases, however, the patient feels calmer and more peaceful after receiving acupuncture.

In certain situations, acupuncture is inappropriate. It should not be performed if the patient is extremely hungry or full, intoxicated, or extremely fatigued. In these cases, the treatment may not be as effective or the person might experience dizziness or exhaustion. People with bleeding disorders such as hemophilia should also avoid acupuncture therapy, although careful application of acupressure or moxibustion is safe. A number of points should not be used during pregnancy due to their tendency to induce labor. Acupuncture is generally not used in children younger than 6 years of age.

HERBAL MEDICINE

Herbal medicine is as old as humanity itself. Early human beings were hunter-gatherers whose survival depended on their knowledge of their environment. Direct experience taught them which plants were toxic, which ones imparted strength and sustained life, and which had special healing qualities. These early discoveries were passed along until thousands of years and millions of human trials brought about the evolution of an incredibly sophisticated system of diagnosis and herbal medicine.

Thousands of medicinal substances are used in China today. Indeed, more than a million tons of herbs are used each year in China. This information may seem astonishing to the minds of Westerners, who see herbal medicine as a newer development in healing. From a practical perspective, however, a fairly complete pharmacy stocks about 450 different individual herbs. From this collection of herbs, a clinical herbalist employs more than 250 standard formulas, each of which can be modified to fit a patient's individual pattern of disharmony.

The herbalist or practitioner combines herbs based on the diagnosis, using a traditional herbal formula as a foundation and adding other herbs specific to the individual's complaint and constitution. As the person's health improves, the nature of the imbalance changes, so the herb formula must also change. Some herbs are deleted when they are no longer needed, while others more appropriate to the changing condition are added.

Herbs are classified according to whether they have a warming or cooling effect on the body. Their taste also has significance. Generally, sweet herbs tonify qi, sour herbs are astringent, bitter herbs dry damp and clear heat, acrid herbs disperse cold and stagnation, and salty herbs have a softening, purging effect. Both individual herbs and herbal formulas are organized into categories, based on diagnostic patterns. For example, if a person has deficient kidney yang, the practitioner selects herbs from the category of "herbs that tonify yang."

The traditional formulas, or patent medicines, are an intricate combination of herbs chosen to address the various aspects of a disease pattern. The *chief* herb in the formula addresses the major complaint; the formula usually contains more of this particular herb than other herbs. The *deputy* herb assists the chief herb in its function, while the *assistant* herb reinforces the effects of the chief and deputy or performs a secondary function. The *envoy* directs the formula to a certain part of the

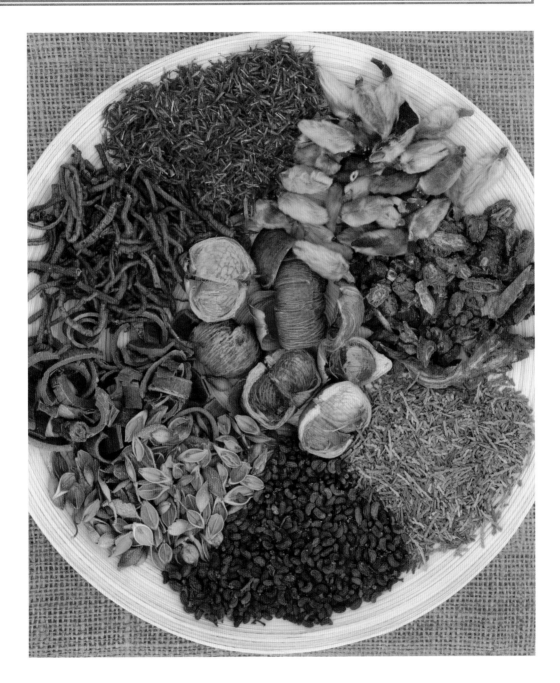

body, or it harmonizes and detoxifies the other parts of the formula. For example, Ephedra Decoction is used for wind cold with wheezing, stiff neck from cold, and a lack of sweating. *Ephedra* is the chief herb, since it treats all of the main symptoms.

Cinnamon twig is the deputy because it assists *Ephedra* in promoting sweating and warming the body. Apricot seed acts as the assistant by focusing on the wheezing, while licorice is the envoy because it harmonizes the actions of the other herbs and restrains the *Ephedra* from inducing too much sweating. Larger formulas may have multiple herbs that produce the different functions, depending on the desired action of the formula.

Herbs can be taken in the form of decoctions, pills, liquid extracts, powdered extracts, and syrups. Decoctions tend to be the strongest medicine, followed by concentrated liquid extracts, concentrated powdered extracts, and pills. All are effective, and the use of the different forms depends on the individual's personal choice. If you don't have the time to make a decoction or you don't like the taste, pills or capsules will be more effective, simply because you'll be more likely to take them. The concentrated liquid extracts tend to take effect quickly, so they are useful in cases where fast action is important, and the syrups are good for sore throats or as tonics. However, many of the more concentrated extracts are available only from a health care practitioner. In whatever form they are taken, though, accurately prescribed herbal formulas are exceptionally effective in restoring health and vitality. This ancient art of traditional herbal medicine is, without a doubt, one of China's great gifts to humanity.

MOXIBUSTION

Moxibustion, or moxa, is named after the Japanese word mokusa, meaning "burning herb." It was first recorded in medical texts during the Song Dynasty (A.D. 960), but it has most likely been in use much longer. It is an important therapy in traditional Chinese medicine; the ancient texts advise that moxa should be tried if acupuncture and herbs have failed to heal the disease. The heat from moxibustion is very penetrating, making it effective for impaired circulation, cold and damp condi-

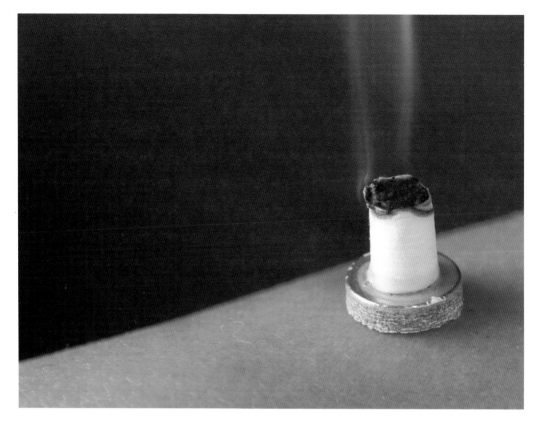

tions, and yang deficiency. When applied to acupuncture points specific for yang deficiency, the body absorbs the heat into its deepest levels, restoring the body's yang qi and "life-gate fire," the source of all heat and energy in the body.

Moxa is prepared from mugwort *(Artemisia vulgaris)*, which is a common perennial herb. The aromatic leaves are dried and repeatedly sifted until they are fluffy.

There are two heating techniques used to apply moxibustion: indirect moxa and direct moxa. In indirect moxa, the "moxa wool" is rolled into a long cigar shape and wrapped in paper. The cigar-shaped moxa stick is then lighted and held about an inch away from the desired area—an acupuncture point or other area of the body chosen by the practitioner. Indirect moxa can be used on acupuncture points to achieve a systemic, or bodywide, effect or it can be used directly at the site of a problem. For example, indirect moxa might be applied to a swollen, stiff area such as an arthritic joint. It is also appropriate to apply indirect heat to specific acupuncture points, such as Zusanli (Stomach 36) or Mingmen (Du 4), to create a systemic effect. The heat taken into these points raises the body's metabolism and immunity, so moxibustion at these points can also be used in preventive health care. One ancient text declares that "one who applies moxa daily to Zusanli (Stomach 36) will be free of the one hundred diseases." Applying moxa to Stomach 36 has an energizing effect on the body, especially in regard to immune and digestive functions. Some indications for its use in Chinese medicine are to treat general weakness, anemia, indigestion, nausea, chronic fatigue, shock, allergies, and asthma.

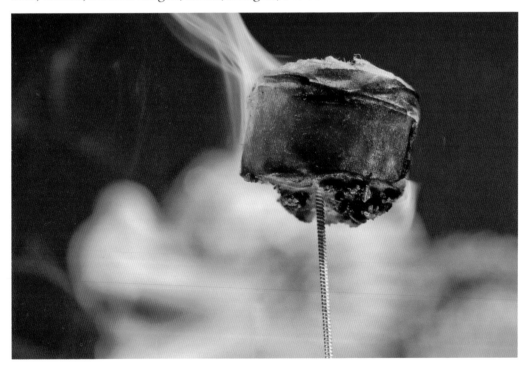

Another type of indirect moxa involves rolling the moxa, placing it on the end of an acupuncture needle while the needle is in the body, and igniting it. The heat from the moxa travels down the handle and into the needle. The needle transfers the heat specifically to the desired point on the body.

In direct moxibustion, a small amount of herb is rolled into a cone and burned directly on the skin. This can sometimes cause a burn, so this technique is rarely performed in Western acupuncture clinics. In most cases when moxa is applied directly to the skin, some ointment is first placed on the point to avoid a burn. In other techniques, the moxa is burned on top of a slice of ginger, garlic, or aconite; this prevents a burn and also adds the therapeutic effects of those herbs to the treatment.

In all cases, moxibustion can be a very pleasant sensation, especially when the warmth spreads through areas that have pain and swelling due to cold. Indirect moxa is also easy to learn to do at home. Practitioners often show a patient the appropriate point for their condition, and the person can take a moxa stick home to perform daily treatments. Such treatment can be very empowering, since the patient then takes responsibility for his own healing.

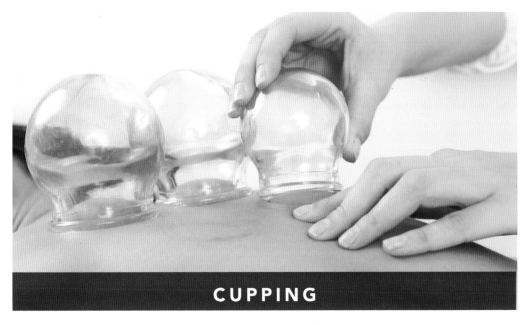

CUPPING

Cupping is a fascinating therapy in which a special cup or jar is attached to the skin by means of suction. The suction is created by heating the air inside the cup to create a vacuum, then quickly pressing the mouth of the cup to the desired area. There are also modern cups that can be applied with a suction device. Interestingly, cultures all over the world are known to use this technique, making it virtually a universal practice. In ancient times, it was done with bamboo cups or animal horns, and it was often employed to treat external conditions of the skin and muscles such as sprains and strains and drawing out pus. It is especially effective for musculoskeletal pain, often relieving the pain after a single application. The force of the suction draws stagnant blood to the surface of the body, sometimes leaving a round bruise in the shape of the cup. Since pain is caused by the stagnation of qi and blood, the goal of this therapy is to remove the stagnation, increase circulation, and allow healing to take place.

Cupping should not be used when the patient has broken skin, skin ulcers, edema, high fever, bleeding disorders, varicose veins, or convulsions. It should also not be performed on the abdomen or low back of a woman who is pregnant. Care needs to be taken to avoid burning the patient with a hot cup; using the cups with the suction device eliminates this potential problem.

EXERCISE

The practice of qi gong is exceptionally common in China. On any given morning, parks all over the country are filled with people of all ages practicing the graceful movements of both qi gong and tai qi. While most people perform these exercises for their own benefit, a practitioner can impart healing energy to a patient's body through medical qi gong methods.

Qi gong (pronounced chee guhng) has been practiced in China in its various forms for thousands of years. It consists of exercises involving specific breathing practices and/or movements, with the goal of enhancing and balancing qi. The central princi-

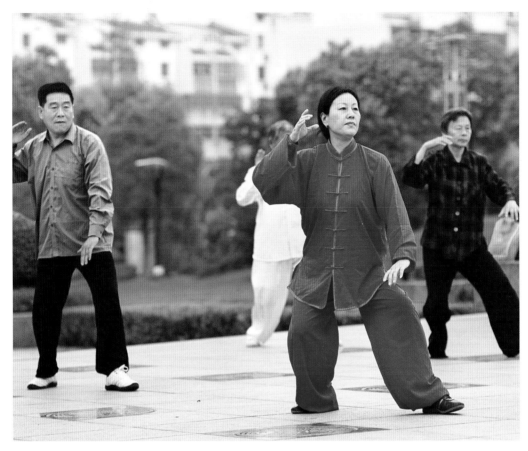

ple involves meditating on a vital energy center known as the Dantian (pronounced dahn tyehn). Located about three inches below the navel, it is considered the root of qi in the body. By focusing on this area while moving the body, a person is able to build up a storehouse of qi and direct it to areas that need it.

Qi gong has a wide variety of forms, ranging from quiet meditative exercises that bring about a sense of peace and well-being to techniques that send powerful waves of energy flowing through the body. In its medical form, qi gong is used to build immunity, treat disease, improve strength, clarify the mind, and enable a person to tap into underlying reserves of energy. The ancient Chinese physician Hua Tuo is quoted as saying "a running stream never goes bad," meaning that qi and blood will not become stagnant if proper exercise keeps them circulating. He developed a set of exercises known as "imitation of five animals boxing," which was an early form of both qi gong and tai qi. He and his followers were able to remain healthy into old age by practicing these exercises regularly.

As Chinese medicine grew more sophisticated over time, the practice of qi gong also became more focused on curing specific diseases. By the 19th century, it was used clinically for ailments such as indigestion, toothache, eye problems, headache, abdominal pain, and chronic degenerative diseases in general.

The practitioner of qi gong trains in order to master three groups of exercises: those that regulate the body, those that regulate the heart and mind, and those that regulate breathing. The purpose of these exercises is for the practitioner to learn to release muscular tension, strengthen the muscles and tendons, and circulate qi and blood to the various organs and regions of the body. Different positions are assumed, depending on the desired result, but in all cases a profound relaxation allows the muscles and organs to rest and rejuvenate. Meditating on the Dantian also allows the practitioner of qi gong to become free of distracting thoughts, bringing about a state of inner peace and heightened awareness. In medical qi gong, it is possible to direct the healing energy to specific organs and meridians. The patient can do this, and it is also possible for the physician to direct healing qi into the patient's body through his or her hands. When qi gong is combined with acupuncture treatment, the therapeutic results can be truly remarkable.

THERAPEUTIC MASSAGE (TUI NA)

No healing modality could possibly be older than massage, since it is such a basic human instinct to rub a painful area. The Chinese have developed a sophisticated system of massage over a period of thousands of years that is used for numerous conditions. Going far beyond the expected applications for musculoskeletal pain, this massage technique is taught in Chinese medical schools, and specialists in the art are able to treat a wide range of diseases effectively. By working with the meridian system, practitioners are able to treat internal conditions such as hypertension, peptic ulcer, insomnia, nausea, arthritis, and constipation.

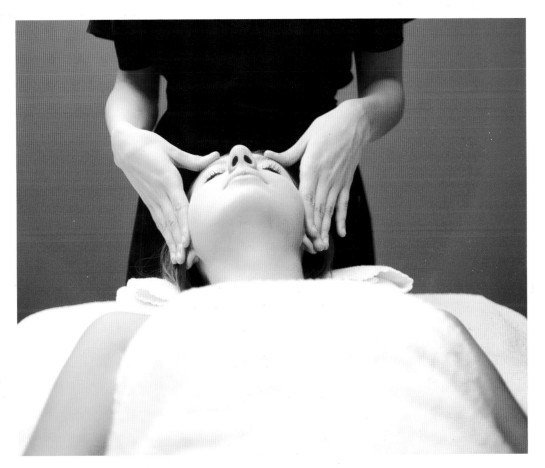

Pediatric massage is a field of specialty practiced in Chinese hospitals. It is especially effective on children younger than 5 years of age, and the younger the child, the more effective the treatment tends to be. The caress of a loving parent is the first sensation a baby experiences after birth, and recent research in the West has shown that infants who are routinely touched tend to be healthier and gain more weight.

Some of the conditions treated by pediatric tui na, or massage, are diarrhea, vomiting, poor appetite, common cold, fever, bed-wetting, and crying at night. As in adult therapeutic massage, pediatric massage involves a variety of manipulations, such as pushing, spreading, kneading, pinching, and pressing. The manipulations are chosen according to the level of stimulation desired and the nature of the area massaged.

The results of Chinese therapeutic massage can often be quite dramatic, bringing about an immediate sense of healing. It is especially effective when used with other modalities, such as herbal medicine. For example, in an injury, herbs are taken internally to reduce the inflammation, swelling, and pain. In addition, a topical herb formula is combined with oil and massaged into the injured area to increase circulation and healing to the area, augmenting the systemic effect of the internal formula. This sort of three-pronged approach ensures a much faster recovery time, and it is one of the reasons that tui na practitioners are held in such high regard in China.

DIETARY THERAPY

Chinese dietary therapy is an integral part of any complete treatment plan. The earliest written record is Sun Simiao's *Prescriptions Worth a Thousand Gold,* published in A.D. 652, in which he discusses the treatment of a variety of diseases through diet. For example, his treatment for goiter included the use of seaweed and the thyroid glands from farm animals. This early iodine and hormone replacement therapy predates Western discoveries by hundreds of years. Similarly, in A.D. 752, Wang Shou published *A Collection of Diseases,* in which he describes his treatment for diabetes. He recommended the use of pork pancreas as a treatment, predating the discovery of insulin by 1,000 years. In the absence of laboratory tests, his method of checking for sugar in the urine was ingenious: The patient was instructed to urinate on a flat brick to see if ants would show up to collect the sugar!

In the traditional system of dietary cures, foods have been organized into categories based on their innate temperature, energetics (the direction in which they move qi and how they affect qi and blood flow), and the organs they affect. For example, a person who has a wind cold condition with excessive clear mucus might be told to consume hot soup made from onions and mustard greens. The onions are warming, expel cold, and sedate excess yin. The mustard greens have similar properties, and they also help expel mucus and relieve chest congestion. Flavoring the soup with ginger and black pepper enhances the warming, expectorant action. With such a lunch, one can imagine that the person's herb formula would be much more effective. On the other hand, if the same patient decided to have salad for lunch with a cold glass of milk, the cold and damp nature of this meal would make the wind cold condition much worse. Any herbal therapy administered at this point would be much less effective, since the therapy first needs to overcome the negative effect of the food before dealing with the acute ailment. For this reason, a patient is always advised about which foods could exacerbate the imbalance and which will help restore balance.

In general, grains and beans are considered to bring stability to the body. They build blood and qi, and they establish rhythm and stability. Vegetables, which are best if eaten in season, bring vitality. Leafy greens have an affinity for the upper body, while root vegetables give strength to the middle and lower body. Fruits build fluids and purge toxins, and they tend to be cooling by nature. They should be eaten alone, or they can cause indigestion. Meats possess the full range of temperatures, and they are a simple source of blood. But they are meant to be consumed in small quantities. Finally, dairy products are a good source of fats, but they should also be eaten in moderation. Overconsumption can result in excess dampness or mucus. A healthy diet should consist mainly of a wide variety of organically grown whole grains, beans, and vegetables; fruits and animal protein should be eaten in smaller amounts.

A TYPICAL TREATMENT PLAN

A practitioner of traditional Chinese medicine may specialize in acupuncture only or herbal medicine only; other practitioners practice both. On its own, each therapy system can effectively treat a wide range of diseases. However, most practitioners agree that a highly effective treatment consists of a combination of acupuncture and herbal medicine. A typical treatment plan might consist of an acupuncture treatment once a week with herbs taken between treatments. This combination of acupuncture and herbal therapy is applied often in the West, where most people must pay out of their own pockets for acupuncture treatments. Using herbal therapy between acupuncture treatments provides continuous treatment at a lower cost to the patient.

Acupuncture and herbal therapy also work in a synergistic fashion, supporting each other. In the case of a knee injury, for example, acupuncture needles are inserted at the site of injury to increase the flow of qi to the injured area. To accentuate the effect, herbs are prescribed that have a general strengthening and anti-inflammatory action. As the inflammation subsides, moxibustion and massage are added to the treatment plan. As the patient's condition further improves, qi gong and tai qi exercises are added to the treatment plan to bring additional strength and qi flow to the area of healing.

There is no typical duration of treatment in traditional Chinese medicine, since each case is treated individually. A person with an acute, but simple, condition might feel completely free of illness and pain after just one acupuncture treatment, while another person with a chronic disorder might require weekly acupuncture and daily herbal medicine for a few months before the condition is rectified. In all cases, however, the practitioner chooses the treatment modality he or she believes will be most effective in view of the practitioner's experience and the individual receiving treatment.

FINDING A QUALIFIED PRACTITIONER

Acupuncture and traditional Chinese herbal medicine have been practiced quietly in Asian communities in the United States for more than 150 years. It remained "underground" as an isolated cultural phenomenon until 1971, when interest was sparked by the experience of *The New York Times* reporter James Reston. His experience of acupuncture in China led him to write an article in which he stated, "I have seen the past, and it works."

Now that acupuncture and traditional Chinese medicine are entering the mainstream of the practice of medicine in North America, an increasing number of people are interested in finding a qualified practitioner. As with all professional services, the best way to find a practitioner is through a referral. If a trusted friend or relative has had favorable experiences with a practitioner, many people will feel safe consulting that physician. In some areas, other health care professionals might provide a referral to an acupuncturist, especially if they work in a holistic group practice.

There are also certifying agencies that establish standards that a practitioner must meet to be considered qualified. The most established is the National Certification Commission for Acupuncture and Oriental Medicine (NCCAOM), established in 1982. After three to four years of training, a student is qualified to sit for a licensing exam. The NCCAOM's extremely high standards for scholastics and clinical training become evident to any student who has been through this rigorous process. NCCAOM certification is used as the basis for licensure in 98 percent of the states that have set standards for the practice of acupuncture.

As with any health care provider, you are well within your rights to call practitioners and ask them about their training and experience. If you have a particular condition, ask them if they have any experience in treating it. It is always important to work with somebody with whom you feel comfortable.

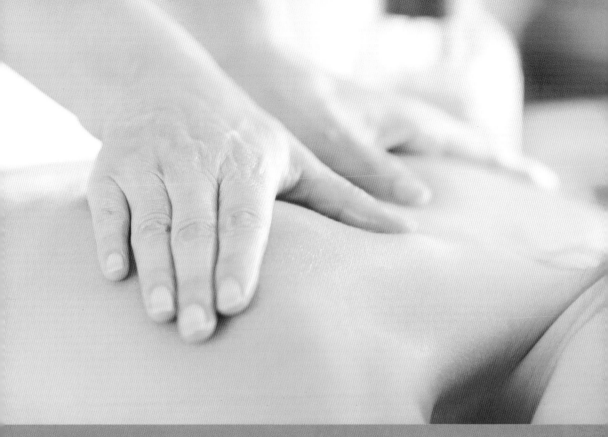

MASSAGE

Not that long ago, the mere mention of massage therapy met with a snicker or roll of the eyes. Many viewed massage as a sleazy activity at worst, a flaky one at best. But in the last couple of decades, attitudes have shifted dramatically. More and more people—of all ages, from all walks of life—are discovering that massage not only feels good, but is good for your health and general well-being.

Massage has gained credibility among traditional medical practitioners, making its way into hospitals and clinics. Many insurance providers have begun covering massage therapy in certain situations, and physicians have begun prescribing and recommending it. There are more than 300,000 massage therapists and students in the United States today!

HISTORY OF MASSAGE

Humans in diverse cultures have used massage for thousands of years as a means to improve health. The ancient Egyptians treated diseases with massage, and for centuries the Chinese have considered massage to be an essential ingredient of their approach to health care.

Modern massage was introduced to the United States in the 1850s by two New York physicians who had studied in Sweden. The first massage therapy clinics were opened here after the Civil War by two men from Sweden. Massage became popular for a while during the 1870s, but public interest gradually faded. Today, however, many doctors advocate the value of massage as useful therapy.

HEEDING HIPPOCRATES

Greek physician Hippocrates advocated massage and wrote that "the physician must be experienced in many things, but most assuredly in rubbing."

MASSAGE AND PAIN RELIEF

Many types of pain have reportedly responded to massage therapy. These include back pain, pain from cancer and cancer treatment, carpal tunnel syndrome, neck pain, fibromyalgia, migraine, muscle strain, rheumatoid arthritis, temporomandibular joint disorder (TMD), tension headache, and whiplash. Massage may also play a role in the prevention of pain. For example, massage can soothe away tension before it triggers a headache, while a post-workout massage may help reduce an athlete's chances of getting sore muscles later on. In addition, massage helps relieve stress, anxiety, and depression, whether these result from illness, injury, trauma, or life's everyday pressures. If you have high blood pressure and have been told you need to relax more, getting regular massages may be a tool you can add to your kit.

How does massage work to relieve pain? One theory is that the pressure from massage closes down the pain gate to the brain, so the pain signals sent by your muscles aren't perceived by your brain. Massage also seems to relax muscular tensions that can trigger pain. And it may improve circulation, reduce stress hormones such as cortisol and norepinephrine, and stimulate the flow of body chemicals that serve as natural painkillers and mood-elevators. People also report that massage helps raise their energy levels and get better, deeper sleep.

WHEN MASSAGE ISN'T A GOOD IDEA

Massage should never be applied to the site of an open wound, injury, cancer, or skin infection. People with a history of blood clots should avoid deep, high-pressure massage techniques that might loosen a blood clot and lead to an embolism. If you have any doubts about whether you have a health condition that would contraindicate massage therapy, talk to your primary health care provider.

TYPES OF MASSAGE

Generally defined, massage is the kneading, stroking, and manipulation of the soft tissues of the body—that is, the skin, muscles, tendons, and ligaments. One question that people have is whether massage will cause pain. It's true that sometimes muscles will ache as they're massaged and tension is worked out, but don't be pressured into a massage that's too intense by thinking, "no pain, no gain." You may also experience some soreness the day afterward, as if you've been working out. Ice can help, as can gentle stretching.

There are dozens of different massage techniques. Here are some of the more common.

Swedish massage. Stroking, kneading, and mild tapping of soft tissues are all part of Swedish massage, which is the most frequently used type of massage in the United States. The therapist uses oil or lotion so his or her hands can move smoothly over the skin. In general, if a spa, gym, or clinic is offering "massage," they're referring to Swedish massage. It's often offered in blocks of 30, 60, or 90 minutes.

Deep-tissue massage. This technique, similar to Swedish massage, utilizes deeper pressure in order to loosen tight muscles. It's considered especially useful for treating chronic conditions. People frequently feel sore after deep-tissue massage, and if you have arthritis or a similar condition, check with your doctor before committing to deep-tissue massage—it may not be the type of massage that's best for you.

Chair massage. You'll see these massages offered in places like airports or hotels. These massages can be a quick way to relieve some stress if you have 20 minutes or so to spare.

Acupressure. An ancient Chinese technique, acupressure involves various hand and finger movements—pressing, pushing, rubbing, squeezing, and the like—on designated areas (acupoints) along the body's meridians. The purpose of acupressure is to open blocked energy channels that result in disease or pain. See the section of acupuncture in the chapter on Chinese Traditional Medicine for further explanation of the philosophy behind this method (see page 26).

Amna and shiatsu. Amna is traditional Japanese massage, based on traditional Chinese medicine. Modern shiatsu, in turn, developed from amna. The term "shiatsu" means "finger pressure," and as with acupressure, fingers and palms are used extensively to manipulate the muscles. Shiatsu is a bit different from the Swedish massage that most Westerners are used to. There is no use of oil, so people do not generally disrobe; it's customary to wear loose, comfortable clothing to a shiatsu massage.

Hot stone massage. Hot stone massage involves placing smooth stones warmed by water on specific points on the body; the heat acts to relax the muscles. Cool stones can sometimes be used for contrast. The massage therapist may also hold the stones and use them to apply pressure.

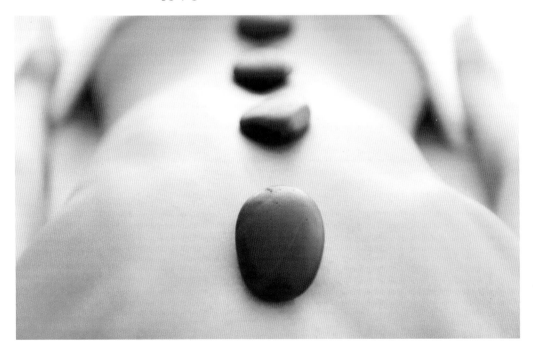

Prenatal massage. Prenatal massage can help expectant mothers relieve aches and pains caused by pregnancy. Therapists work with their clients in order to make them comfortable and use positions that are safe for mother and baby. Women with high-risk pregnancies should, however, consult their doctor or midwife before beginning a massage program.

Geriatric massage. Massage can be very helpful for older patients, especially those who suffer from common conditions like high blood pressure or arthritis. In general, the practitioner will use a lighter, gentler touch for older clients.

Reflexology. Reflexology is massage that focuses on the feet, although the hands are sometimes also involved. Specific points on the feet and hands are thought to be reflex areas for other parts of the body, including the glands and organs. The therapist applies pressure to these spots, both to diagnose what's wrong and to stimulate healing of the corresponding body part. See page 59 for more on reflexology.

Sports massage. Specifically tailored for the athlete, sports massage focuses on parts of the body that get frequent use in a particular sport. For example, the legs of a cyclist and the arms of a swimmer get special attention. Massage before athletic activity helps warm up the muscles, while a post-workout massage seems to stimulate blood circulation and clear away lactic acid residues that cause muscle soreness.

Thai massage. A Thai massage therapist not only applies pressure to various parts of the body, but stretches the body. A Thai massage can look a bit like someone helping someone else achieve a yoga pose! It's meant to increase flexibility and range of motion. Wear loose, comfortable clothing to a Thai massage.

Trigger-point therapy. Trigger points are sensitive spots in the muscles that are often painful. They result from repetitive motions, injuries, accidents, or other types of trauma. Over time, disease and aging can increase the painfulness of sensitive trigger points. Deep pressure applied to these areas brings about pain relief. For chronically irritable trigger points, several sessions may be needed to completely clear the problem.

FINDING A MASSAGE THERAPIST

You can often find a massage therapist through referrals from friends or health care providers, or by reviews on Yelp or similar web sites. You can also check the web site for the American Massage Therapy Association (amtamassage.org)

Before an appointment, confirm that your prospective massage therapist is licensed to practice in your state and does the type of massage you're interested in. (Most, though not all, states regulate massage therapists.) If you're not sure what type of massage would be right for you, talk about any problems you're having, any health conditions you have, and what your goals are in order to get guidance. If you're getting a massage at the recommendation of your doctor or after an injury, check your insurance to see if they cover massage therapy (and what limits apply) and check with the clinic or spa to confirm that they take your insurance. Ask them if there are any forms you will need to fill out when you arrive, or that you should fill out in advance—many clinics will have an intake form asking about your general health, any medications you're on, and so forth.

You may also want to ask beforehand about tipping guidelines—in the U.S., it's generally customary to tip in spa settings, but not always when you're going through a medical practice.

FOOD AND DRINK

In general, it's recommended that you don't eat heavily before a massage. Do, however, stay hydrated, both before and after your massage. Many massage therapists will offer you a glass of water after your session as a standard practice.

At the session itself, discuss the problems you want to alleviate and what areas of the body you'd like the therapist to focus on. A good massage therapist will work with you to make the experience comfortable, productive, and relaxing. Throughout the massage, the massage therapist will probably check in with you on your comfort level. Don't be afraid to ask questions or to check in with the therapist if something feels wrong or even just less than optimal. Here are some things to consider:

- **Would you like more or less pressure to be applied?**

- **Are you experiencing unexpected pain?**

- **In a hot stone massage, are the stones too hot for comfort?**

- **Is the room too warm or too cold?**

- **If music is playing, is it too loud or distracting?**

- **Do you have any scent allergies or sensitivities that mean that certain oils or lotions are not for you?**

With some types of massage therapy, such as Swedish massage, it's usual to disrobe to some level so that oil can be applied. The therapist should respect your comfort level, leaving you alone to remove clothing and, throughout the session, draping a sheet or covering over the parts of the body that aren't being worked on.

A therapist who pushes you to disrobe further than your comfort level, who doesn't listen to your needs, or who talks during the session if you ask for silence, is not the massage therapist for you! Don't be afraid to speak up yourself if something seems off!

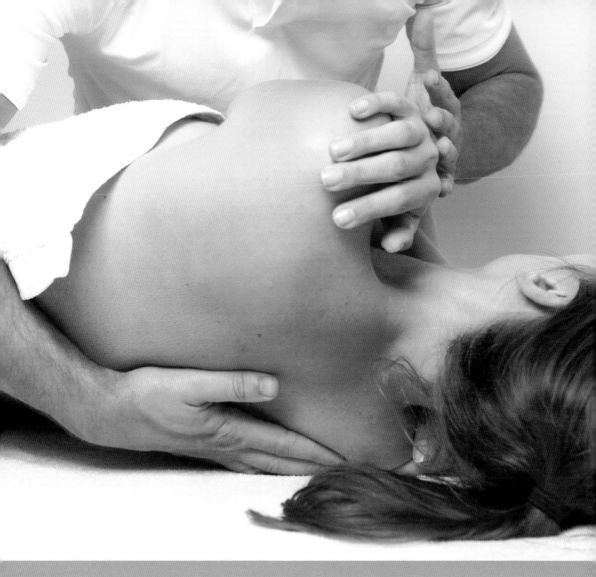

CHIROPRACTIC

Native Americans, the ancient Chinese, the South American Incas, and many other people throughout history have used spinal manipulation of one form or another to combat pain and illness. Probably the first physician to proclaim the benefits of spinal adjustment was Hippocrates, the Father of Medicine himself, when he advised his students, "Get knowledge of the spine, for this is the requisite for many diseases."

MODERN CHIROPRACTIC

Daniel David Palmer, a Canadian who later settled in Iowa, is credited with starting modern-day chiropractic. Palmer had a long-time interest in natural healing, which he finally pursued professionally. The healing technique that eventually became known as chiropractic originated one September day in 1895 when a janitor was explaining to Palmer how he'd lost his hearing 17 years before. He had exerted himself while in an awkward position and felt something in his back give way. The story piqued Palmer's interest, and he convinced the janitor to let him try a spinal adjustment. After several adjustments, the man regained his hearing.

Today, with more than 50,000 active practitioners in the United States, more and more people are turning to chiropractors than ever. It's one of the most popular of all alternative therapies. Many insurance companies and health organizations have indicated their support of chiropractic by including it in their benefit plans.

VOCABULARY TIP

The term chiropractic was devised by the Reverend Samuel Weed, who was one of Palmer's patients. Weed took the term from the Greek words for "hand" and "practice."

WHAT IS CHIROPRACTIC?

Chiropractic's focus is the spine, which acts as a communication center for the body's nervous system. Because the nervous system connects to every part of the body, chiropractors see it as the key to overall health. Misalignments in the spine (historically called subluxations by chiropractors) put pressure on the nerves, thus interfering with normal nerve function. The result: pain and illness. The theory is that freeing the spine of subluxations, through spinal manipulation of adjustment, will restore health.

Although some people associate chiropractic with body-cracking procedures, many types of chiropractic therapies exist today. A practitioner may use one or a combination of the following methods:

- **A common technique that gently stretches a joint slightly beyond its normal range of motion. Often this causes a cracking or popping noise, which is attributed to a release of gases from joint fluid.**

- **A gentle-touch technique, which does not involve forceful adjustment and does not produce cracking sounds.**

- **A hand-held instrument with a rubber tip that gently moves vertebrae into alignment.**

- **Network chiropractic, or network spinal analysis, is a gentle technique that relies on a specific sequence of adjustments.**

Historically, there have been two broad categories of chiropractic practice, traditional and mixed. Practitioners of traditional chiropractic focus only on spinal manipulation. "Mixed" chiropractors, who are more common these days, mix several techniques, and may blend other natural health care therapies such as massage, nutrition and lifestyle counseling, exercise, and heat or cold treatments into their practice.

DOES A SPINAL ADJUSTMENT HURT?

A spinal adjustment may leave residual soreness, comparable to muscles that have been worked through exercise. Any pain should go away after a day or two at most.

WHAT CAN CHIROPRACTIC DO?

Although many people associate chiropractic with fixing a bad back, some practitioners claim chiropractic treatment has achieved excellent results in treating many ailments. The relief of back pain, especially lower back pain, has been studied the most in clinical research. For evidence of the use of chiropractic to treat other conditions, people tend to rely more on anecdotal evidence that suggests that the treatments are helpful. Some of the conditions that have been said to benefit from chiropractic are allergies, arthritis, asthma, bladder infections, the common cold, diabetes, ear infections, gastrointestinal disorders, headaches, high blood pressure, menstrual problems, peripheral joint injuries such as in the hands, elbows, and shoulders, poor vision, respiratory problems, sexual dysfunction, sinusitis, sleep disorders, and sports injuries.

The American Chiropractic Association web site notes that, "Chiropractic care is used most often to treat neuromusculoskeletal complaints, including but not limited to back pain, neck pain, pain in the joints of the arms or legs, and headaches."

Not only do some chiropractors advocate use of their healing techniques to "fix" the body when it's out of balance, they also recommend chiropractic for prevention of health problems. The theory is that a well-aligned body is better able to stave off disease and dysfunction in the first place.

COMPLICATIONS AND CAUTIONS

Sometimes serious health problems, not directly treatable by chiropractic, can manifest themselves as back and neck pain. These include cancer, endometriosis, osteoporosis, ulcers, and other problems. Your doctor and chiropractor should help you evaluate whether your back or neck pain has origins that are suited to chiropractic adjustment. They can advise you whether you need another type of medical treatment instead or in addition to chiropractic.

CHOOSING A CHIROPRACTOR

Chiropractors go through an extensive four-year academic program to obtain their doctor of chiropractic degree (D.C.). Then, before setting up a practice, they must complete a written examination covering multiple topics besides chiropractic per se (anatomy, hygiene, pediatrics, physiology, physiotherapy, X-rays, and more), plus a practical exam that assess their clinical capability and techniques.

Consider the following pointers when choosing a chiropractor:

- **Get a recommendation from your primary health care provider. You can also ask trusted friends who have had chiropractic treatment for the health problem for which you want to get treatment. The American Chiropractic Association's web site is also a good resource.**

- **Contact your state chiropractic examining board to find out if any disciplinary actions have been filed against a particular practitioner and whether he or she is properly licensed.**

- **Find out what type of chiropractic therapy is practiced.**

- Be wary of anyone who presents chiropractic as a cure for every problem. If the chiropractic tries to talk you out of seeing your doctor or seeking other health care advice, walk away.

- As with any practitioner, ask how many years the person has been practicing and how much training and experience does he or she have.

Once you've begun treatment:

- Remember that overexposure to radiation from X-rays can pose health risks, so be alert to the frequency of X-ray procedures, and don't hesitate to ask questions about them.

- If you haven't noticed any change after a few weeks of chiropractic, it may be wise to look into another type of treatment.

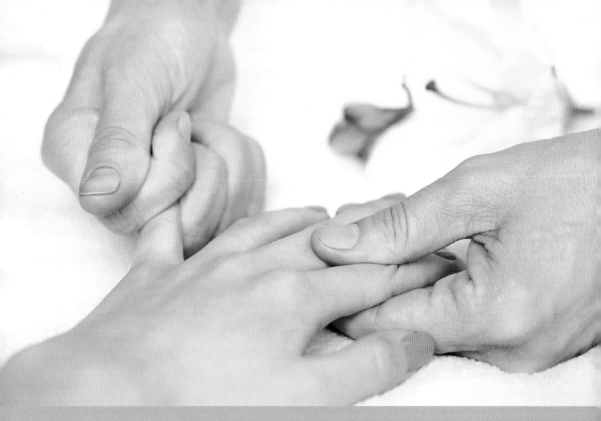

REFLEXOLOGY

The practice of reflexology involves application of pressure to regions on the feet, hands, and ears, the idea being that each region is connected to a corresponding gland, organ, or system of the body. Does this feel good the way a massage feels good? Absolutely. Can reflexology reduce stress? Again, yes, but it doesn't stop there. One of the theories underlying reflexology takes matters a step further in its faith that the body can and will repair itself if given a reprieve from stress. Specifically, reflexologists believe that applied pressure, by reducing stress, affects the correlated organ or system and can reduce pain, improve circulation, enhance the quality of sleep or relaxation, and reduce psychological symptoms such as anxiety and depression. For example, reflexology correlates a specific spot in the arch of the foot to the bladder; reflexologists maintain that by applying appropriate pressure to this area, bladder functioning is positively affected.

REFLEXOLOGY IN HISTORY

The origins and history of reflexology are not easy to track, but the practice is thought to have been passed down through oral tradition. Reflexology was first recorded as a pictograph, along with other medical procedures, in 2330 B.C., on the Egyptian tomb of a physician named Ankhmahor. The scene is a raised relief, and depicts men manipulating the hands and feet of others.

The Huangdi Neijing, an ancient Chinese medical text also known as *The Yellow Emperor's Classic of Internal Medicine,* is dated by scholars to between the late Warring States period (475–221 B.C.) and the early Han period (206 B.C.–220 A.D.), and contains a chapter on "Examining Foot Method." This work, a summation of Chinese medical knowledge up to the time of the Han dynasty, is written in the form of a dialog between the semi-mythical Yellow Emperor, Huang Di, and various ministers. It marks the beginning of discussions in print about the connection of life force to specific points and areas on the body.

Reflexology and massage traveled to Europe courtesy of Marco Polo, who is credited with translating a Chinese massage book into Italian in the 1300s. The ideas caught on: it is said that in the sixteenth century the Florentine sculptor Cellini made a practice of pressing on his toes and fingers to relieve pain elsewhere in his body. In 1582, European Doctors Adamus and A'tatis published a book about zone therapy, the holistic idea that a body's cells and organs make up an interactive organism; this concept was to become the basis of modern reflexology. Around this same time, Dr. Ball of Leipzig, Germany, published a booklet in which he discussed the treatment of organs via pressure points.

It's said that President Garfield applied pressure to his feet to relieve pain, but the idea of zone therapy didn't really gain traction in the United States until the early twentieth century, thanks to an ear, nose, and throat doctor named William H. Fitzgerald. In 1917, Fitzgerald, who is often referred to as the father of reflexology, wrote about ten vertical zones that extend the length of the body. Fitzgerald described discovering how pressure applied to one part of the body could deaden pain in other areas. This led him to map out various areas and their associated connections, and note what conditions could be influenced through manipulation of these areas.

Decades later, American physiotherapist Eunice Ingham developed Fitzgerald's ideas further: she diligently created even more detailed maps of the feet, drawing on her experiences working with hundreds of patients. She is credited with discovering that an alternating pressure is more effective than continuous pressure, and with creating the "thumb walk" technique discussed below. Her first book, *Stories The Feet Can Tell,* was first published in 1938; the text, which documented her cases and described in detail the energy zones of the feet, propelled her into 40 years of lecturing and teaching on the subject of reflexology. Today Ingham is considered a pioneer of the field.

LET A MAP BE YOUR GUIDE

Foot maps or charts guide practitioners— who can include physical therapists, massage therapists, and chiropractors— as they apply pressure to specific areas. The maps, with their careful labeling and bright colors, demonstrate the detail and interest of a good medical illustration and illustrate which parts of the foot correlate with certain parts of the body. Examine one of these maps, and you'll see that though our left and right feet share many characteristics (the toes on either foot are connected to the sinuses, for example), they are not mapped as mirror images of one another. The left foot corresponds to the organs and valves found on the left side of the body, and the right foot to all organs found on the right side. A spot on the heel of the right foot correlates to the appendix, for example; the pressure point for the spleen, by contrast, exists on the left foot only.

DIFFERENT FROM A FOOT MASSAGE

Reflexology is sometimes confused with foot massage, but the two are very different practices. Foot massage, a close cousin to Swedish massage, typically incorporates massage oil or lotion and involves gentle gliding strokes all over the foot; essentially, massage is a systematic working of the soft tissues of the body to release tension, a sort of "working from the outside in." It's an enjoyable process, and while reflexology can also be pleasant, as noted above, reflexologists focus on specific points in the feet, hands, and ears. They believe that manipulation of these areas directly benefits other, corresponding parts of the body by releasing congestion or stress in the nervous system— in other words, they are "working from the inside out."

In "thumb walking," the most common technique used in reflexology, the therapist uses the edge of her thumb in an inchworm motion; she moves along taking small "bites" out of the area she works upon. Reflexologists may also use rubber balls, rubber bands, and sticks of wood to assist their practice.

WHY DO PEOPLE GET REFLEXOLOGY TODAY?

Ingham's work prompted curiosity and allegiance; years later, reflexology is regarded as a useful complement to more traditional medical practices. Even staunch supporters of Western medicine have conceded that reflexology may aid in the reduction of pain, and be useful as part of palliative care for people with cancer. Reflexologists also work with clients seeking relief from stress or fatigue. Patients burdened by a heavy workload (and attendant side effects) have credited reflexology with restoring energy levels and helping to achieve a calmer attitude; it is argued that this improvement then puts clients in a position where they might better manage their challenging schedules.

And perhaps that is the underlying beauty of the practice: some things—work schedules, stress, illness—can't be avoided. But reflexology can help clients manage those conditions, often in concert with other practices (e.g., reflexology is not considered a substitute for medical care), and in so doing allow them to live their best lives.

WHAT YOU CAN EXPECT

What can you expect during a reflexology session? Typically, the practitioner will begin by conducting a brief health and lifestyle history. He or she will ask about what illnesses have been previously diagnosed, recent operations, and if you are currently taking medication or herbs, then ascertain whether reflexology is indeed a good choice of therapy for your needs (for example, reflexology is not recommended during the first trimester of pregnancy, and certain conditions such as osteoporosis require a modified approach). The practitioner will explain how reflexology works, and what you can expect during the session. He or she should make clear that the practice does not cure specific illnesses, and should not be considered a substitute for medical treatment. You may be asked to sign a consent form.

Depending on your specific health needs, the reflexologist will proceed with work on the hands, feet, ears, or some combination of the three. Some situations dictate the approach taken; if a hospital patient is hooked up to multiple IVs, for example, the reflexology session may be limited to more accessible areas, like the feet.

If the reflexologist works on your feet, you will be asked to sit or lie down. You can expect to remain dressed except for your shoes and socks; the reflexologist may wash your feet or soak them in warm water before positioning them at chest level.

Before beginning the session, the practitioner will check your feet and hands for wounds, rashes, sores, warts or bunions, and ascertain if you have any pain that should be accommodated during treatment. If you have a specific health concern, the practitioner will keep it in mind during the therapy, carefully feeling and working the area corresponding to the ailment. But whether you suffer from migraines or are battling sciatica, the reflexologist will also work other areas on the hands or feet with a gentle, settled pattern, beginning at the toes (or fingers), working down to the heel of the hand or foot, then manipulating the areas on the sides and top and, in the case of the feet, working to the knees. Pressure should be firm but not painful.

Reflexologists usually work on one foot at a time. If the practitioner encounters congestion, tightness, or pain during the session, he will work that area to bring the body back into balance. Reflexologists do not claim to "fix" the pain themselves; rather, they believe that they are stimulating the nervous system to do the work. If your practitioner finds a trouble spot, he may return there at the end of the session, to confirm that pain has abated.

People receiving reflexology often report physical and emotional responses to the treatment, including a sense of relaxation and rest, tingling in the body, or feelings of warmth. Reactions may also include perspiration of hands or feet, coughing, laughing, a sensation of light-headedness, or the desire for sleep.

Sessions typically last 30 to 60 minutes. You can rest or talk during the session; some people actually fall asleep! Practitioners should be present and grounded. Some play relaxing music during treatment, or burn aromatic oil or candles, and many close the session with a calming action such as stroking the hand or foot in a comforting manner. After your session, the reflexologist may suggest that you drink water to help flush toxins from your body, rest if necessary, and pay attention to your body during the next few hours. It is also recommended that for approximately 24 hours after treatment, you avoid stimulants like coffee, and eat light meals.

IS REFLEXOLOGY RIGHT FOR ME?

The effects of reflexology are unique to each person. Many report a sense of relaxation and well being after treatment, but some individuals have experienced less pleasant after-effects, including:

- **Nausea**

- **Cold-like symptoms**

- **Lethargy**

- **Tiredness**

It is a good idea to consult with your general practitioner before pursuing reflexology treatment if you have existing health concerns or are taking medication for a condition.

CHOOSING A REFLEXOLOGIST

If you decide to move forward with reflexology, do careful research before choosing a practitioner, as you would when looking for any doctor or healing practice.

Watch out for practitioners who:

- **Are evasive or dismissive of your questions and concerns.**

- **Rush the practice or rush you after the session concludes.**

- **Claim that reflexology treats specific illnesses or is a substitute for medical treatment.**

- **Are lay practitioners, perhaps trained at a massage school or two-week course, and who lack the in-depth training required for reflexology certification.**

A good practitioner will:

- **Answer your questions.**

- **Conduct a brief health history prior to session work.**

- **Take the time to explain how reflexology works and what happens during a session.**

- **Have received the proper training. Preferably, you will work with a nationally certified reflexologist who has trained at an accredited institution and passed a national board exam (note that most nationally recognized programs require 110 hours of reflexology training).**

- **Have some experience: it takes a lot of practice to build responsiveness in the fingers and awareness of energy flow.**

- **Have pursued continuing education courses since receiving their certification.**

Don't hesitate to reach out to family and friends for recommendations. People who have first-hand experience with a practitioner—and who know you—will have valuable input. It's worth it to take the time to find a reflexologist who feels right for you.

REFLEXOLOGY FOR ANIMALS

Some people embrace the concept of reflexology for their beloved cat or dog friends. Adherents claim that humans and animals share similar anatomy, physiology, and health concerns, and possess identical energy centers (chakras) and energy pathways (meridians) in their bodies. The thinking is that humans and animals alike accrue stress during daily life; why wouldn't similar practices alleviate that stress?

The practice of animal reflexology identifies important energy points on the paws, similar to the reflex points on human hands and feet. The cat map, for example, connects the tips of the paws to head and neck, and the pad to chest and abdominal organs. The inner edge of the paw relates to the spine. Some practitioners have noted that while dogs prefer touch to their back paws, cats are more comfortable with work on their front paws. Stroking the ears, particularly the tips, is believed to alleviate stress and anxiety.

Most people agree that when we engage with our animal friends with love, stroking their ears or petting their backs, we can see how they benefit; we hear the purr, we see the love in their eyes. Just by touching an animal, we help them. What may not be completely understood is how powerful touch can be to an animal's overall health.

Of course, as is the case with humans, pet reflexology should not be a substitute for conventional medical practices; rather, reflexology should be considered a complement to regular veterinary care.

REFLEXOLOGY AND WOMEN IN LABOR

Reflexology is gaining currency as a simple, inexpensive, and noninvasive technique to help women in labor: with pain, with labor duration, even with the baby's APGAR scores. Some studies have concluded that reflexology, when used as a complementary alternative technique, reduces labor pain intensity because touching and skin contact help reduce stress. The evidence suggests that because stress and pain are connected, with stress worsening pain and pain worsening stress, less stress during labor can lead to less pain.

Less stress or anxiety during labor leads to other positive outcomes. Because less anxiety is associated with lower adrenaline levels, and because high adrenaline levels can disrupt uterine muscle activity (and thus increase labor length), proponents believe reflexology, by easing stress, can help reduce the duration of labor.

Finally, some studies have pointed to reflexology as contributing to higher APGAR scores. The APGAR score, typically assessed at one minute and five minutes after a baby's birth, is a simple measure of how a newborn is doing (APGAR stands for Appearance/Pulse/Grimace response/Activity/Respiration). Points are assigned to each category, and a higher score is desirable; the assessment helps determine if a baby requires additional medical assistance. Continuous pain and fear in a labor affects a mother's systems, including respiratory and circulatory; when the body is adversely affected, a more difficult labor can result, which is in turn harder on the baby and drives down the APGAR score. Reflexology, with its calming properties, has been linked to easier labor and higher APGAR scores.

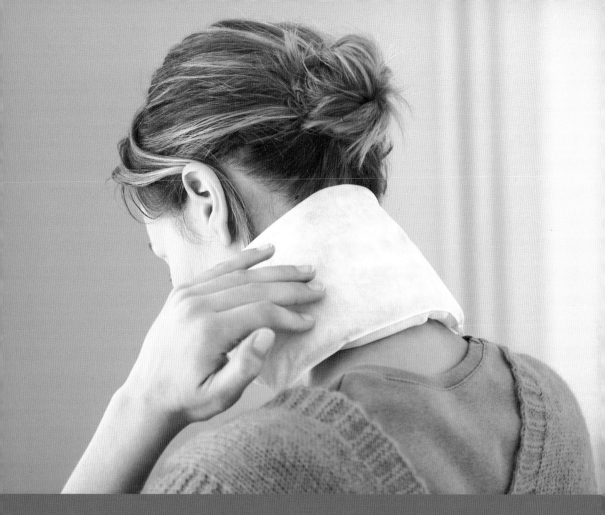

COLD AND HEAT TREATMENTS

Throughout history, humans have used cold and heat to ease pain and discomfort. From Native-American sweat lodges to Scandinavian saunas, people have used heat to relieve tense muscles and stiff joints, as well as to boost general well-being. Cold has been used to treat painful injuries since Hippocrates used ice and snow back in the fourth century B.C. Today, modern medicine still relies on heat and cold to relieve many painful conditions.

USING COLD

There are many forms of cold treatment for pain relief. The most common are ice packs, ice massage, cold compresses, immersion in cold water, or evaporative sprays that leave a cooling after-effect. Commercial ice packs are available, but a bag of crushed ice wrapped in a towel also works well in a pinch. Refreezable gel packs offer the advantage of being flexible, so they conform better to the shape of the injured area; a bag of frozen peas will do the trick, too.

Whatever you use, be sure there is no direct contact between the ice and the skin. If possible, hold the ice pack in place with an elastic bandage (not too tightly), which will compress the injured area. If you injure a hand or foot, it may be better to immerse it in ice water rather than apply an ice pack. For an Achilles tendon, put two socks on the injured foot, then stuff a plastic bag filled with crushed ice between the socks to cover the painful area.

MUSCLE AND JOINT INJURIES

Ice is an inexpensive, highly effective treatment for such injuries as sprains, pulled muscles, bruised shoulders, and torn ligaments. Certain types of chronic pain, such as tendinitis and bursitis, also respond to ice treatments. For any of these conditions, ice is most effective when it is applied as soon as possible after the injury or the onset of pain. That's because ice reduces swelling and tissue damage, promoting faster healing. Studies have shown that prompt icing can cut recovery time by as much as half.

How long you should ice for depends on the injury. It's commonly advised to treat an injured area for 10 to 20 minutes. For an area with many nerves close to the surface area, you probably don't want to ice for more than 20 minutes at a time.

After the initial application, apply ice every couple of waking hours for the next 48 to 72 hours. If swelling or pain returns later, apply ice again.

RICE FOR RELIEF

When you suffer a sprain, strain, pulled muscle, or torn ligament, remember the acronym RICE for a treatment routine:

- REST to help soothe the pain and avoid making the injury worse.

- ICE the injured area immediately.

- COMPRESS the injured area to reduce swelling by wrapping it with an elasticized bandage, but be careful not to wrap too tightly.

- ELEVATE the injured area to above heart level to help reduce swelling.

OTHER WAYS TO USE ICE

Some experts recommend using an ice pack to relieve headache pain. Apply ice either directly to the area where you can feel the pain, or place it on the back of your neck. You can also try an ice hat, a special type of ice pack that surrounds part of the head.

Many people recommend an ice massage for shin splints, which are small tears in the muscle attachments on the sides of the shin. The easiest way to do this is to freeze a paper cup filled with water, then peel back the cup's rim so you can rub the ice up and down on your shin muscles from knee to ankle.

Similarly, you can use ice massage for painful heels by rubbing them with a plastic jar filled with ice or by rolling your heels over an ice-filled jar.

COLD COMPRESSES

While some experts recommend ice packs for headaches, some people find cold compresses more effective and comfortable. For a tension headache, a cold compress placed against the back of the neck may help. For sinus headaches, apply a cold compress to the forehead and the area below your eyes and above your upper jaw, where sinus cavities are located. Make a cold compress by soaking a cloth in ice water and then wringing it out.

CAUTIONS WITH ICE THERAPY

Follow these guidelines to prevent injury from ice therapy:

- **Don't put the ice pack directly on your skin. Wrap it in a thin towel to avoid nerve or skin damage.**

- **Remove the ice for a while when your skin becomes numb.**

- **Check a refreezable gel pack or chemical ice pack occasionally for punctures, as the chemicals inside may burn your skin. Be aware, too, that these kinds of packs can be colder than ice, so you may not be able to tolerate them on your skin as long.**

- **Avoid ice treatment altogether if you're hypersensitive to cold, if you have poor circulation, or if you have any condition that reduces your ability to sense cold.**

- **If you rest while icing, set an alarm or be sure someone is nearby to wake you in case you fall asleep. This will prevent you from inadvertently leaving the ice on too long.**

- **Don't put ice directly on open wounds or blisters.**

- **See your doctor if you fail to see improvement in a day or so.**

COLD THERAPY FOR BURNS?

It can take just an instant: A harried cook grabs the pan of burning food out of the oven or a cup of hot coffee tumbles down over the side of the table, and you have a burn to treat.

Many burns are minor and can be treated at home. The injured skin turns red; that's known as a first-degree burn. Sometimes, tiny blood vessels may be damaged and may leak fluid, causing swelling and a weepy appearance. If blisters appear, the burn is classified as second degree. In third-degree burns, blisters do not form, and the skin turns white instead of red. Don't look to the degree of pain you feel to determine how bad the burn is; deeper burns often hurt less.

There are times when first-aid methods at home just won't be enough. Get medical attention immediately if you have burns on your hands or face or over a joint, like the elbow, if your burns blister or you suspect that you have a third-degree burn, or if you've suffered chemical or electrical burns, where the damage may occur beneath the skin's surface. Consult your doctor before applying any products to burned skin.

For minor burns, gently run cool water over the burned area, use cool compresses, or place the area in a bowl of cool water. The water should be cool, but not ice-cold. Don't run the water full force, as that may cause more injury to the skin.

And note that just because cool water is good for a burn doesn't mean ice is better. It actually restricts the flow of blood, which you want to avoid.

USING HEAT

Heat can alleviate the pain from such conditions as abdominal cramps, arthritis, fibromyalgia, and menstrual cramps. In the case of muscle or joint injury, however, heat is only applied after the injury has been treated with ice for at least 48 hours. Once the swelling is down, heat can be applied to promote healing. At that stage, heat induces greater blood flow, which washes waste products away from the injured area. It also relaxes muscles, prevents spasms, and reduces joint stiffness. If pain or swelling starts to reappear, switch back to ice.

Some physicians recommend foregoing heat treatments altogether. Instead, they suggest alternating icing with moderate exercise sessions. The latter has the same effect of improving blood flow and enhancing healing, and it does so better than heat. Continuing ice applications keeps swelling and pain at bay.

TYPES OF TREATMENTS

Heat treatments can be dry, such as a heating pad or heat lamp, or moist, such as a hot bath or a hot compress. Both dry and moist heat seem to be about equally effective. Health care providers don't all agree on which method is best, but they do agree on one point. Avoid high temperatures. Whether you're applying a heating pad or immersing yourself in a bath, the temperature should feel comfortable to your skin.

In addition to treatments you can do at home, heat treatments are also available through physical therapy or in other medical settings. Whirlpool baths provide immersion therapy. Dipping or immersing a painful joint in paraffin wax can bring relief for such conditions as arthritis. Ultrasound can be used for deeper healing, such as for deep joint pain or fibrous scars.

CAUTIONS WITH HEAT THERAPY

Remember, any external heat treatment should be at a temperature that's comfortable to your skin. Don't overdo it.

Avoid heat treatments if you have circulatory problems or any condition that impairs your ability to sense heat: The risk of getting burned may outweigh the advantages of heat therapy.

Pregnant women need to be especially cautious in avoiding baths that are too hot. Raising the body temperature above 100 degrees Fahrenheit for a long period could result in miscarriage or birth defects.

HEAT FOR FROSTBITE?

Frostbite occurs when the fluids in the skin tissues begin to freeze, or crystallize, restricting blood flow to the affected area. Most cases of frostbite occur on the hands, feet, toes, nose, and ears. The reason is that as the body temperature drops in reaction to prolonged exposure to cold, the heart attempts to protect vital organs by increasing circulation to the torso at the expense of the extremities. The sooner you notice the symptoms of frostbite, and the faster you take measures to rewarm the areas, the better the outlook for recovery. The skin may first start to tingle, as ice crystals begin forming in the tissues. Then, pain develops, accompanied by redness, burning, itching, and swelling. If exposure to cold continues, numbness sets in, the pain decreases, and the skin becomes whiter and waxy looking. At this stage, immediate action is necessary to prevent gangrene, or death of skin tissue.

While it is wise to have any suspected case of frostbite checked out by a doctor, you need to take steps right away to rewarm and protect the affected areas.

If you become frostbitten, don't run to the nearest radiator, hot stove, or roaring fire. You don't want to risk burning tissues that are already damaged. For the same reason, do not use a heat lamp, hot-water bottle, or heating pad to warm up. Submerging the affected extremity in a sink or basin full of warm water (104 degrees Fahrenheit to no more than 110 degrees Fahrenheit) is the safest way to treat the frostbite. Once your fingers or toes are warmed up, very gently wiggle them to increase the circulation to the area. For frostbitten ears or a frostbitten nose, simply staying in a heated room may be enough to warm them sufficiently. If not, gently apply warm compresses to the affected area; do not rub the delicate tissue.

HEAT, COLD, OR BOTH?

For some types of pain, the debate continues as to whether heat or cold is better. For example, heat has been a traditional treatment for lower back pain, but today some people question whether heat is truly the most appropriate treatment for the problem.

Still, individual preferences must also be considered when making therapy choices. After all, a major part of effective therapy is making the patient comfortable enough to continue with the process and ultimately to experience relief.

Sometimes therapists recommend alternating hot and cold treatments in what is known as contrast therapy. Contrast therapy has been used for chronic ailments such as arthritis, TMD, and tendinitis. However, contrast therapy should only be used when ice has brought down any initial swelling.

Finally, avoid using either heat or cold treatments for gout, even though it seems like one or the other would offer relief. In fact, heat increases circulation to the area, and cold may cause more crystals to form in the joint, tendon, or ligament. Either way, you'll end up with more swelling and pain.

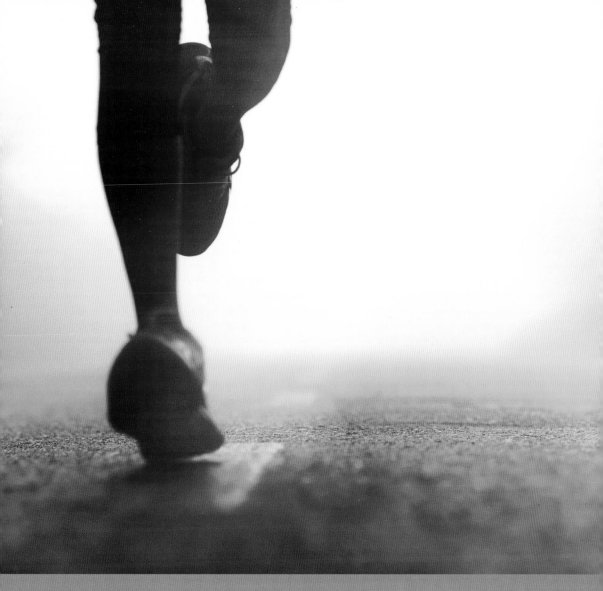

EXERCISE

Today, many of us lead a lifestyle that's more sedentary than that of our ancestors. That lack of exercise can have serious consequences—we need exercise to keep our heart, muscles, and lungs healthy. Study after study shows that regular exercise can reduce the risk of heart attack and stroke, help people manage conditions such as prediabetes and diabetes, and even play a part in maintaining good mental health.

FROM THE ANCIENT TEXTS

In traditional Chinese medicine, there is an understanding that too little exercise can lead to stagnation of qi and blood, and subsequently, a variety of diseases. Some of the traditional Chinese ideas about lack of exercise are expressed throughout the ancient texts:

- **"Sleeping or lying down too much hurts the qi." When a person oversleeps, he or she typically feels tired all day.**

- **"Too much sitting hurts the muscles." This refers to the fact that lack of exercise causes the muscles to atrophy.**

- **"A running stream doesn't go bad." Stagnant water easily becomes spoiled; stagnant blood and qi lead to many different illnesses.**

In fact, the importance of exercise shows up in many ancient medical texts. Hippocrates reportedly said, "Walking is man's best medicine." The famous 10th century physician Ibn Sina (Avicenna), too, wrote of the role of exercise in promoting health. Throughout history, there has been a consensus that exercise helps us maintain our physical and mental health.

SETTING UP A SUSTAINABLE EXERCISE PROGRAM

So how much exercise is necessary? Currently, the American Heart Association recommends that people engage in 150 minutes a week of moderate activity or 75 minutes of moderate-to-vigorous activity. Ideally, people wouldn't go more than a day or two without exercising—so exercising 30 minutes, 5 times a week, will provide more benefits than exercising for hours at a time, once a week. However, anything is better than nothing. If you've been sedentary and want to incorporate more exercise in your life, it may be better to start small and build up.

WHAT ACTIVITIES ARE BEST?

The most important question when you're deciding whether an activity belongs in your program isn't how many calories it burns or how healthy it is. It's whether you'll do it. Set yourself up for success by incorporating things you enjoy—or, at a minimum, activities you don't dislike—in your exercise routine.

If you've been inactive for a while, this can be difficult. Sometimes you need to think outside the box, to activities you haven't thought of as exercise. Do you like to dance, but you only do so at weddings? If so, now's a great time to check out a social dancing class through your local park district or community center. Maybe you find the idea of a treadmill boring, but you like bird watching or admiring architecture—if you do, think about adding in more nature hikes or walks through historic neighborhoods.

And don't be afraid to try something new. You might find that you enjoy the elliptical machine much more than the treadmill, or that you get a kick out of using a rowing machine. If you're competitive in other arenas, you might find that you can apply that competitive drive to games of tennis or racquetball.

BUILDING IN VARIETY

You've no doubt heard the aphorism that variety is the spice of life. It's also the key to a sustainable exercise program. You want to build a program with different types of exercise activities. That way, you won't only exercise the same muscles and joints. Having several potential activities to choose from can also keep you from getting bored and cutting your exercise time short.

Think about the weather—don't rely on activities that can only be performed in good weather. Even if you get a gym membership, incorporate some activities that you can do at home, so that you're not reliant on a working car to exercise. If you travel a lot, look into things you can do on the road.

Different types of exercise will also provide different health benefits. Some activities improve cardiovascular health. Some examples of good aerobic activities include cycling, walking, running, dancing, rowing, and swimming. These are all activities that engage large muscles in repetitive movement and raise your heart rate and breathing for an extended period of time.

Cardiovascular, or aerobic, exercise will tone your muscles, strengthen your heart, improve blood flow throughout your body, and help improve your blood sugar levels. But it won't necessarily do much to make your muscles bigger (if you're a man) or denser (if you're a woman). Adding muscle requires strength training, such as weight lifting. And strength training has its own health benefits. It helps turn fat into muscle, and that improves your basal metabolic rate.

Your basal metabolic rate refers to the calories your body burns just to keep your heart beating, lungs breathing, eyes blinking…in other words, just to keep you alive. This calorie expenditure is like the interest you earn on a bank account: It's essentially something you get for doing nothing but being there.

Fat is metabolically stagnant. In other words, fat cells require virtually no calories to stay alive. Muscle, on the other hand, is very active metabolically. Muscle cells chew through a lot of calories even when they aren't moving. The more muscle you have, the higher your basal metabolism and the more calories your body burns all the time—even when you're resting.

Strength training involves moderate to high exertion for short periods of time. When a muscle is worked to near (but not quite) exhaustion, the muscle becomes stronger and more efficient. Stronger and more efficient muscles burn more calories every minute of the day, whether you are actively working them or not, and they can help you achieve your weight loss goals more quickly.

Other types of exercise will improve flexibility and balance; these are especially good as we age.

WALKING FOR HEALTH

Walking is so simple that we often overlook it as a form of exercise. But it has a lot of advantages. You don't need fancy gear or equipment. It's low impact. And you can fit a brisk 10-minute (or longer) walk into your way of life more easily than almost any other kind of exercise.

Although not as strenuous as jogging, walking will increase your heart rate and oxygen consumption enough to qualify as an aerobic exercise. When you walk, your heart starts to beat faster and move larger amounts of oxygen–rich blood around your body more forcefully. Your blood vessels expand to carry this oxygen. In your working muscles, unused blood vessels open up to permit a good pickup of oxygen and release of carbon dioxide. These changes improve your ability to process oxygen. Better circulation to your leg muscles can mean less leg fatigue and fewer aches.

The aerobic benefits aren't the only ones you'll get by incorporating walking into your life. Walking can refocus your attention from whatever is troubling you, reducing anxiety, tension, and stress. It helps you relax and recharge your mind and body.

DEALING WITH ACHES AND PAINS

When some part of your body hurts, your first inclination may be to lie down and not move a muscle. While that can be appropriate when you first suffer an acute injury, it's precisely the wrong thing to do for other pain, such as chronic back pain, headaches, or arthritis. Remaining sedentary in those cases only makes matters worse.

Indeed, the more medical researchers learn about the body's response to pain, the clearer it becomes that exercise is a key factor in pain management. What's more, exercise can often prevent the onset of pain in the first place by improving physical conditioning, which makes us less susceptible to the stresses, strains, and injuries that can result in pain.

No matter how carefully you exercise, you probably will experience a few little aches and pains—simply because you'll be asking your body to do things that it might not have done for years. Don't let a few minor physical discomforts discourage you. At the same time, don't persist in thinking that you should exercise until it hurts, or work through pain. Pay attention to your body.

Even people who have been exercising regularly complain of occasional soreness and stiffness. The pain may occur immediately following the activity or after some delay, usually 24 to 48 hours. Often the discomfort lasts for only a few days. It is practically impossible to completely avoid muscle soreness and stiffness. But you can reduce the intensity of the pain by planning your conditioning program so that you progress gradually, especially during the early stages. That approach will allow the muscles of the body to adapt themselves to the stress placed on them. If you become sore and stiff from physical activity, doing some additional light exercises or general activity will often provide temporary relief.

MUSCLE CRAMPS AND SPASMS

When one of your muscles contracts powerfully and painfully, you may have a muscle cramp. The contraction may occur at any time—at rest as well as during activity. Cramps usually occur without warning.

Among the causes of muscle cramps are fatigue; cold; imbalance of salt, potassium, and water levels; and overstretching of unconditioned muscles. You can reduce the chances of muscle cramps by maintaining a proper diet, making sure you warm up properly prior to vigorous activity, and stopping activity before you become extremely fatigued.

If a cramp does occur, it can usually be stopped by stretching the muscle affected and firmly kneading it. Applying heat and massage to the area can restore circulation. If you're plagued with frequent cramps, drinking adequate fluid and eating foods with salt and potassium, along with muscle strengthening and stretching exercises, will usually eliminate the problem.

FROM THE EAST

Many Westerners have been discovering the stress-reducing and pain-relieving benefits of exercise methods from across the ocean.

Qi gong and Tai Chi Chuan are centuries-old Chinese exercise forms. Adherents believe that qi gong stimulates and balances the qi, or life energy, flowing through the acupuncture meridians. Tai Chi has been described as "meditation in motion." Its slow, gentle movements are reported to be helpful in releasing tension and relieving pain. For instance, Tai Chi-based exercises are approved by the Arthritis Foundation to help relieve arthritis pain.

Yoga, from India, is another of the world's oldest health practices that has the effects of elevating mood, reducing tension and fatigue, and putting people in a positive mood. We'll look more in depth at yoga and India's traditional medicine in the following chapter.

HOW TO DO A SIMPLE QI GONG EXERCISE

The first step in performing a qi gong exercise is to locate the Dantian, a major energy center in the body near the solar plexus. The point is located below the naval at a distance equal to the width of four fingers. The acupuncture point located there is called "Gate to the Original Qi," and the Dantian is located inside the abdomen about a third of the distance between that point and the spine. This is the focus of meditation during qi gong exercises.

While performing qi gong, it's most important to relax and be calm. Sitting on the floor cross-legged or with legs extended, shoulders relaxed and hands facing down in your lap, meditate on the Dantian as you inhale normally. Continue focusing on your Dantian while you exhale normally, then slowly lean forward and slide your hands out in front of you on the floor. You should be fully stretched out by the end of the exhale, not forcing either the stretch or the breathing. Gradually sit up to the original position as you inhale, continuing your meditation on the energy center. Repeat for a few minutes, then discontinue the focused meditation and sit still with your eyes closed, breathing normally.

After a qi gong session, people typically feel energized and relaxed, ready to deal with the stresses of the world in a calm and grounded manner.

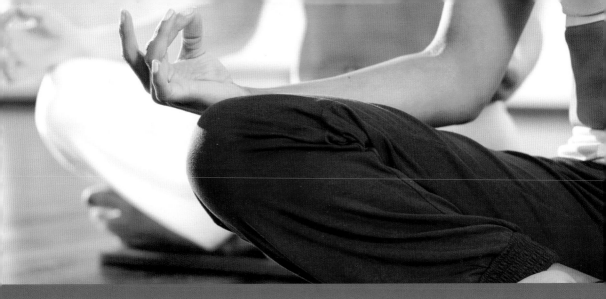

TRADITIONS FROM INDIA: AYURVEDIC MEDICINE AND YOGA

Ancient India is one of the few places in the world that developed a coherent medical system whose tenets remain in practice today. Ayurvedic medicine is still practiced throughout the Indian subcontinent and is enjoying a burgeoning popularity in the West.

In the ancient Indian language Sanskrit, Ayurveda means "the science of longevity" and is sometimes translated more broadly as "the science of life." The system seeks to restore harmony and balance to the body, mind, and spirit through a system of diet, herbal medicine, massage, purification, and lifestyle discipline.

In Ayurvedic medicine, the patient is active in his or her own preventative therapy and restoration. In this sense, Ayurveda is much more concerned with health than with disease—with the healthy person rather than with the unhealthy patient.

Although one of the features that makes Ayurveda so popular today is its "holistic" approach, the truth is Ayurvedic medicine is firmly grounded in empirical observation and scientific theory.

THE ORIGINS OF AYURVEDA

Scholars of Indology cannot determine the exact origins of Ayurveda, but we can see how many different traditions combined to create it over the millennia. The magical, religious lore of early Indian civilizations, the more empirical and practical approach of the so-called wandering ascetics, the medical traditions of the early Buddhist monks, and possible additions from neighboring traditions all work together to provide the basis of what we know as Ayurveda.

Out of these traditions emerged a system eventually codified in the two great Ayurvedic medical treatises—*Caraka Samhita* and *Susruta Samhita*. Although these two works, which provide the basis for the entire system, are considered Hindu, the information in them clearly developed over the centuries with significant help from the Buddhists and other religious and secular traditions.

EARLY BUDDHIST INFLUENCES

About the middle of the 5th century B.C., many Buddhist ascetics—monks and nuns—began to organize into spiritual communities called sanghas. Membership in these sanghas was open, and the monks encouraged other wanderers to seek shelter there, especially during the rainy season. Visiting ascetics, eager to debate and exchange information, brought new ideas and healing strategies, which they debated with apparently great devotion.

As the sangha population stabilized, the monks and nuns began to standardize and codify all the medical information they had gathered. The ancient texts on medicine represent the earliest form of Buddhist healing and closely parallels some of the information that would later be set down in the *Caraka Samhita* and the *Susruta Samhita*.

The Buddha identified the causes of disease as falling into one of the following categories:

- **change of season**
- **past actions (karma)**
- **unusual or excessive activities**
- **violent, external actions (being robbed or attacked)**

These Buddhist healers believed that humans represent or reflect the whole of nature. In other words, humans are microcosms of the universe, containing the same elements that make up all of creation. These elements—space (or ether), air, fire, water, and earth—are combined into three biological forces, or doshas, in humans—vata, pitta, and kapha.

- **Vata is space and air.**
- **Pitta is fire and water.**
- **Kapha is water and earth.**

The doshas came to be seen as responsible for all the functions of our bodies and minds. (They are often called "humors" because of the similarity between this system and the biological understanding of the ancient Greeks who recognized four humors.) English has no adequate translation for the word dosha. Although you'll often see them referred to as air, fire, and water, respectively, or (less delicately) wind, bile, and phlegm, the concept of the dosha is more than that; for example, vata has windlike qualities, but it is not simply wind.

The Buddhist canon, and later Ayurvedic medicine, views disease as a disruption of the doshas. Each dosha has its own seat, where it naturally resides in the body. Disruption of the dosha—its migration to, and accumulation in, another part of the body—will cause illness. For example, if vata is unseated from its seat in the lower bowels and moves to and accumulates in, say, the joints, arthritic symptoms may appear. It would be, therefore, the job of the medical practitioner to evaluate the problem and prescribe a treatment to rid the joints of excess vata.

Each one of these doshas by itself and in combination with the others is vital to the health of the body. Without vata, for example, kapha and pitta could not move. Kapha, which is part water, keeps vata from fanning the fire of pitta out of control and burning up the bodily tissues. Without pitta's fire, the digestive process in the body could not take place.

Each person is made up of a unique combination of vata, pitta, and kapha. This combination, created at conception from the combined doshic makeup of one's parents, is called the prakriti, or constitution. To preserve good health, a person must maintain the same ratio of doshas he had when he was conceived.

By understanding a person's doshic makeup, a physician can help anticipate potential problems before they arise and more accurately assess the nature of an illness when it occurs.

RULES OF CONDUCT—
PRACTITIONER AND PATIENT

Both the Buddhists and the early medical treatises (the *Caraka Samhita* and *Susruta Samhita*) map out a physician's code of ethics not unlike the Greek Hippocratic Oath. The Buddhist doctrine insists that the monk-healer be competent, kind, and generous, never refusing medical care to anyone.

The *Caraka Samhita* reminds the physician to be current in his medical knowledge, never betray his patient's trust, "pray each day for the welfare of all beings...and strive with all your heart for the health of the sick." In the *Susruta Samhita*, physicians must be intelligent, have practical experience, and hold fast to the principles of satya (truth) and dharma (duty). Their attendants must give affection to the patient, never grow tired, and carry out the wishes of the physician.

THE DEVELOPMENT OF AYURVEDA

By the first few centuries A.D., Hinduism was ascendant in India. Buddhism found adherents to the east in Tibet and China, and Hinduism absorbed a great deal of theology and science from the Buddhists.

In medicine as religion, the Hindus incorporated what they valued from the Buddhist tradition into their emerging system. Elaborating on earlier concepts and finally codifying what was probably common, orally transmitted knowledge, Indian physicians were finally setting down the tenets of Ayurveda.

The *Caraka Samhita* and *Susruta Samhita,* the sacred medical texts, represent the first true codification of the Ayurvedic system. The *Caraka Samhita* is primarily a clinical medical text; the *Susruta Samhita* is primarily a surgical text. The Samhitas make up the basis of Ayurveda and are still considered authoritative on many issues today.

Diagnosis takes on a much different meaning in Ayurveda than it does in Western medicine. Western physicians seek to identify disease after it produces symptoms; Ayurvedic doctors prefer to monitor the body before illness is manifest. They pay attention to the interaction between wellness and illness, between order and disorder. This way, when an imbalance occurs in the body, the doctor can more easily detect its nature and administer the proper treatment.

DIAGNOSING DISEASE

For thousands of years, Ayurvedic healers have relied on their keen powers of observation and their knowledge of the interactions of micro- and macroanatomy to diagnose disharmony in the body. Through an elaborate interview process, urine and feces analysis, and observation of the tongue, skin, eyes, nails, and other physical features, Ayurvedic doctors can determine which doshas, tissues, channels, and organs are affected. To find the disturbed dosha, a physician needs to establish the patient's individual prakriti (constitution). Like any good doctor anywhere, an Ayurvedic physician takes into account a patient's mental and emotional condition as well as the physical.

When diagnosing an illness, according to the *Caraka Samhita*, a physician must take into account the following items:

- **patient's condition**

- **family background**

- **heredity and caste (social class)**

- **climate, food, and water in the country of the patient's birth**

- **character and temperament**

- **physical constitution**

- **whether the disease is hot or cold**

The *Caraka Samhita* also specifies the proper physical examination, which should include:

- **general appearance of the patient**

- **the feel of the patient's skin (checking temperature)**

- **examination of eyes, tongue, feces, and urine**

- **tasting the secretions of the patient, when appropriate**

Since all disease stems from a disruption in the doshas, treatment must begin to return the body to a state of doshic harmony. Ayurvedic physicians use diet, herbs, and cleansing techniques to counteract the manifestation of disease in the body.

Ayurveda believes it is vital to eliminate the toxins that are causing the disease before attempting to pacify or temper the body. The reasons are simple: First, if a doctor prescribes a treatment that merely attends to the superficial symptoms of an ailment, the disease may go further into the tissues and move away from the treatment. So while the symptoms may get better temporarily, in the long run the disease will manifest elsewhere in the body, causing further debilitating symptoms. Second, an accumulation of undigested foods or toxins (ama) prevents the body from absorbing the herbs and foods designed to treat the disease.

TREATMENTS

There were and are several primary means of treatment to prepare or tone the body. To eliminate disease from the tissues, Ayurveda uses a two-step approach: palliation and purification. In a way, palliation therapy is similar to the Western-style approach called detoxification and cleansing. Purification therapy, however, goes beyond the Western understanding of elimination. Ayurveda believes no treatment can successfully eliminate the toxic wastes from the body without first directing these toxins to their proper channels of elimination. If disease manifests in the body because of an imbalance in the gastrointestinal tract (the first stage of disease), an Ayurvedic physician will almost always perform purification therapy. If the disease has already entered the tissues, however, palliation techniques must precede purification.

YOGA

Most Westerners' conception of yoga is of people meditating in the traditional lotus position and reciting a mantra. While this image is not entirely incorrect—yoga does involve meditation, poses, and sometimes mantras—it is a rather limited picture. Yoga is much more.

Although yoga is not a "healing" system like Ayurveda or traditional Chinese medicine, it strongly encourages and promotes the good health of its practitioners for higher purposes. To combine and advance body, mind, and spirit, humans need health, enlightenment, and inner peace. To this end, yoga uses a psychological and physiologic system to gain control of and exercise both the body and mind, thereby freeing the spirit.

Yoga sees health as a state of bodily harmony that cannot be taken for granted and, as such, demands serious discipline. Falling ill usually denotes a false relationship to one's life and to other people. Feeling ill at ease or alienated from society contributes to creating disease in the body. To return to good health, a yogin must return to a moral and happy life, understanding his or her interconnectedness to all beings. And it cannot be denied that yogic disciplines impart great health benefits to its practitioners.

From ancient times the practice of yoga has sought to deliver its practitioners from the cycle of birth, death, and rebirth that characterizes many Indian worldviews and lead them toward self-realization and ultimate liberation. To attain enlightenment, the yogin (male) or yogini (female) had to strive to keep the body as healthy and as strong as possible through a successive series of techniques, which include postures, breathing, and meditation or contemplation.

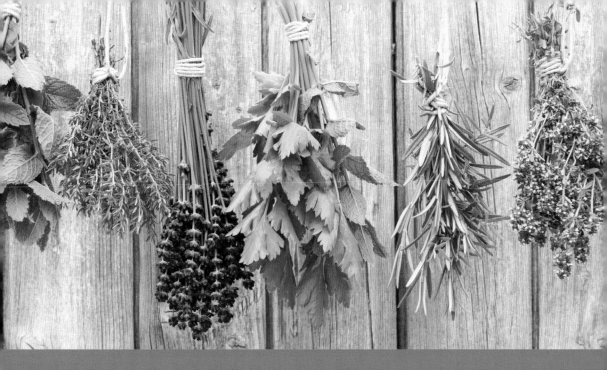

HERBS FOR HEALTH AND HEALING

Herbs have long intrigued us—and for good reason. Because of their potential as food and as medicine, they have enjoyed a special relationship with humans throughout the ages.

To our ancestors, knowledge of herbs meant survival. But the passage of time did not diminish human beings' respect for the herb. Druids revered the oak and mistletoe, both rich in medicinal attributes. In the Eastern world, physicians wrote tomes on herbal remedies, some prized to this day as authoritative medical sources. Later, the Greeks and Romans cultivated herbs for medicinal as well as culinary uses. Hippocrates, considered the father of Western medicine, prescribed scores of curative herbs and taught his students how to use them. The search for precious herbs and spices led Europeans to the New World. There they found scores of new plants that they brought back with them to the courts of England, Spain, and France.

The development of pharmaceutical drugs some 100 years ago changed our focus from herbs and natural healing to the new "wonder drugs." Medical practice turned away from botanicals and embraced these new chemical-based medicines. In addition, the Industrial Revolution meant urbanization, and city dwellers, who now had limited access to gardens, welcomed the convenience of shopping for—instead of growing—their medicines and foods.

In recent years, however, herbs have enjoyed a renaissance. Though lifesavers in countless cases, pharmaceutical drugs proved not to be the magic bullets we'd hoped for. Seeking ways to feel better without the side effects of pharmaceutical drugs, countless people are rediscovering herbs as natural remedies. What exactly is an herb? No group of plants is more difficult to define. In general, an herb is a seed-producing plant that dies down at the end of the growing season and is noted for its aromatic and/or medicinal qualities. Among the most utilitarian of plants, herbs lend themselves to a seemingly endless array of medicinal preparations. And you don't have to be a pharmacist—or a shaman—to make them.

Like other healing traditions, herbal medicine recognizes and respects the forces of nature: Health is seen as the proper balance or rhythm of natural forces while disease is an imbalance of these forces. Because the forces of nature are not easily grasped and manipulated, herbal traditions turn to the earth's masters of natural balance and symmetry—plants.

Indeed, plants are ideal biochemical medicines. We have built-in systems for metabolizing plants and using their energies. But our bodies have difficulty metabolizing and excreting synthetic chemical medicines. And think about the negative terms used to describe the actions of synthetic pharmaceuticals: they suppress, they fight, they inhibit. They do little to support overall health. Medicines made from plants, on the other hand, tend to nourish the body without taxing it, to support the body system rather than suppressing it.

ANCIENT HERBAL MEDICINE

It was our ancestors, in their search for nourishment, who uncovered the roots of medicine. The Neanderthal and Paleolithic peoples were hunters and gatherers who lived intimately with nature, using plants as food, clothing, shelter, tools, weapons, and medicine. They discovered certain plants could optimize their health while others reduced fertility or made them ill. As they learned which plants were not poisonous, which were nourishing, and which were palatable, they also noted which could calm a nauseous stomach, ease the pains of childbirth, and heal wounds. Some Stone Age artifacts appear to be tools that could grind grains, roots, seeds, and bark—early precursors of the mortar and pestle we use today.

Ancient India and Ayurvedic Medicine (about 10,000 B.C. to present): Some of the oldest known writings are clay tablets unearthed in what is now the Middle East. Many of these ancient clay tablets mention healing plants. Within these early writings are four books of classic wisdom, called the Vedas, from which the system of Ayurvedic medicine, as well as the Hindu religion, arose. Ayurvedic medicine looks to nature as the source of wellness, thus its use of healing plants. An Ayurvedic doctor or herbalist begins by identifying which dosha type(s) an individual is; this allows him or her to use an herb with a corresponding physiologic action.

Ancient China and Taoism (5000 B.C. to present): Ancient Asian cultures also embraced the idea that one should seek a balance with the natural forces within all life forms. Chinese Toaism embraces a bipolar medical system rather than the tripolar system of the Ayurvedic doshas. The life force is seen as the ever-churning circular motion of two opposing actions, yin and yang. All diseases are understood as an imbalance of yin and yang. All matter, including plants and animals, is yin and yang (although one usually dominates); therefore, plant qi can be used to balance animal qi. A disturbance in a person's qi may affect the balance of yin and yang. For example, if qi is blocked, yang may predominate. Some herbs are predominantly yin tonics, some are yang tonics, and most are a complex combination of yin and yang. Chinese herbalists must be familiar with each plant's energy to prescribe the herbal remedies with the most healing potential.

Ancient Egypt (4000 B.C. to 1000 B.C.): The Ebers papyrus is one of Egypt's most important surviving medical writings. Dating from approximately 1550 B.C., this 65-foot papyrus scroll was discovered in 1873 by Georg Ebers, a German Egyptologist. The document includes both herbal and medical therapies, including numerous substances still thought to be medicinally active, such as garlic and moldy bread. The Egyptians had a sophisticated knowledge of plants, as their practice of using myrrh in embalming attests.

Ancient Greece (1000 B.C. to A.D. 100): The Iron Age witnessed the flourishing of civilization. During that time, the first medical schools were formed, foreign lands were explored, and goods were traded. One of the medical schools founded in Alexandria emphasized the study of poisonous plants. Some of the most prominent physicians were:

- Crateuas, who lived about 100 B.C., was a plant collector and herbalist for King Mithradates VI, known as The King of Poisons. The drawings by Crateuas are the earliest known botanical illustrations. His was the first illustrated pharmacopoeia, which classified the plants and explained their medicinal uses.

- Pendanius Dioscorides, a Greek who lived around A.D. 100, served as a physician to the Roman army. He traveled extensively throughout Europe and published the five books commonly referred to as *De Materia Medica*.

A compendium of nearly 600 plants, it was the leading pharmacologic text for 16 centuries. This thorough work included most of the previously existing herbal literature.

- Hippocrates, considered the Father of Medicine, believed in gathering data and employing observation and experiments in his practice and study of medicine. (He helped commence the Age of Reason.) Hippocrates banished magic, superstition, and incantations. Instead, he embraced the life force, the laws of nature, the body's innate ability to heal itself, and the healing power of nature—all principles that relate to herbalism. He stated, "Nature heals, the physician is only Nature's assistant."

- Galen, a Roman physician, authored an astounding 400 books, half of them on medical subjects, including *De Simplicus*, an herbal. He created potent medicines by combining plant, animal, and mineral substances.

Arabia (A.D. 800 to present): The Arabian physician Ibn Sina (Avicenna) is credited as the first to distill essential oils from aromatic plants. One of his books, the five-volume *Canon of Medicine,* an authoritative and monumental compendium of all medical knowledge at the time, remained in use in Europe for more than 700 years from its publication about A.D. 1020.

Europe in the Elizabethan Era (Late 1500s to Early 1600s): The Swiss physician Paracelsus lived from 1493 to 1541. Paracelsus traveled throughout Europe studying chemistry, alchemy, and metallurgy and their application to medicine. He reasoned that plants had some sort of active chemicals that were responsible for their actions. Because Paracelsus wrote in the common language of the people rather than in Latin, he was lauded by folk healers, and, likewise, Paracelsus respected them.

An English apothecary, Nicolas Culpeper sought to remove power from medical doctors and put it in the hands of the apothecary profession. He supported educating people to care for themselves—especially those who could not afford doctor visits. He disturbed the entire medical profession by translating the *London Pharmacopoeia* from Latin to English in 1649, putting it in the hands of the common people. Culpeper is also known for his association with the Doctrine of Signatures, an ancient concept that held that the physiologic action of a particular plant on the human body can be learned or inferred from observing the plant and getting to know its character and appearance.

John Gerard, an Englishman who lived around the same time as Culpeper, was a barber-surgeon. In those days, many physicians dispensed medicine only. Barber-surgeons filled the gap by offering minor surgical procedures. The red and blue striped barber pole is a remnant of the old symbol used by the barber-surgeons—the blue stripe represents venous blood and the red stripe represents arterial blood. And yes, you could also get your hair cut while you were undergoing surgery. Gerard published the *General History of Plants*, more commonly known as *Gerard's Herbal,* in 1597.

Early American Medicine: The medicine of early Americans was a blend of Native American remedies and numerous European traditions. The early settlers brought seeds and plants with them from Europe to the new land; some native American plants, such as plantain, dandelion, and red clover, were already familiar to them. Many households had a family herbal—held in nearly equal esteem with the family Bible—to which they often referred during times of illness. As the colonies grew, the new Americans learned from each other and the Native Americans, incorporating the practices of the different cultures into their medical knowledge.

GETTING STARTED

Herbalism in the United States has been undergoing a renaissance since the early 1970s, with the reemergence of the naturopathic medical profession after its decline in the 1950s and 1960s. Research dollars are increasingly becoming available to investigate botanical therapies. Nurseries stock a wide assortment of culinary and medicinal herbs. Public seminars and symposia on herbal medicine are often filled to capacity.

The recent interest in herbs and herbal medicines has led to a boom in herbal products. A whole gamut of herb types and strengths is now available, and there's a variety of ways to use and consume them. With so many herb products available, you may not know where to start. But don't despair: Anyone can learn how to use the most common herbs—safely and easily.

You can purchase herbal medicines at your local health food store or natural-product pharmacy. You can also make herbal remedies yourself, which is a less expensive—and very satisfying—alternative.

BUYING HERBS FOR HOME USE

When buying a bulk herb for use as a cooking spice or tea, or for making your own homemade herbal products, choose herbs with a strong aroma, color, and flavor. Selection is fairly easy once you become familiar with an herb's characteristic odor, taste, and appearance. Many grocery stores carry fresh culinary herbs in the produce department, and health food stores and specialty herb stores carry dried herbs in bulk bins or jars.

Compare an herb's characteristics in preparations, too. If an herbal tea imparts a strong color to the water, with a good aroma and strong flavor, its quality is probably good. Teas and tinctures with pale colors and weak flavors are of poor quality. If possible, select teas that have been harvested less than one year ago. Look for tinctures made from fresh plants.

You will most likely want to start with the inexpensive, grow-your-own or readily available herbs. Be sure to begin with herbs considered entirely nontoxic. However, note that "safe" and "nontoxic" do not mean 100 percent reaction-free; they do mean nonlethal and almost always harmless. Individual reactions can occur from any substance, including mint, garlic, or alfalfa.

CAN HERBS BE DANGEROUS?

When using any herbal remedy, educate yourself about the herbs you're interested in. Do not take any substance unless it is indicated for the problem you have. Do not assume an herb is safe because it's available in a health food store. Though most products are safe, some may have been formulated with only a rudimentary knowledge of herbs and could prove harmful. Consult a physician or herbalist if you have any questions about the herbs you wish to use or the condition you wish to treat.

Consulting a naturopathic physician or herbalist is absolutely crucial if you use prescription medications. Blood thinning medications, in particular, may interact with herbs, other drugs, and even some foods and are the drugs most often responsible for hospitalization due to adverse side effects. Children and the elderly may require lower doses of herbs.

Always use caution when using an herbal medicine for the first time—don't take handfuls of capsules or drink pots of tea. Begin with 2 to 3 capsules or 1 to 2 cups of tea daily for a few days to see how your body reacts. People who have a history of reacting to prescription drugs or people who are very sensitive to perfumes or soaps should be cautious. For any serious or persistent health complaints, you should consult a naturopathic or other type of physician.

Herbal teas and essential oils from an herbalist are likely to be much stronger than their grocery store counterparts. Even common spices an herbalist dispenses, such as cinnamon or ginger, are likely to be of stronger color, flavor, and smell than the cinnamon or ginger in your spice rack. But as interest in herbs grows, fresh herbs and specialty teas of good, strong quality are becoming more accessible to the general consumer.

In general, an herb's potency as a flavoring is intimately linked to its potency as a medicine, and the two actions are likely to diminish equally with time. This is because much of an herb's medicinal actions are due to essential (volatile) oils— the oils in herbs we cherish as aromatic and flavoring substances. As the flavor and aroma wane, the medicinal activity wanes concurrently.

Dried and powdered herbs remain at full potency for about a year. Most tinctures and essential oils maintain a good, strong potency for three to five years.

BUYING HERBAL PREPARATIONS AND ESSENTIAL OILS

When buying herbs in capsule or tablet form, it's often impossible to assess the quality of the herbs. Naturopathic physicians, herbalists, or individuals who have used the product are good sources of information. It's a good idea to do some careful study about the herbs you are considering. Make sure they are indicated for the condition you wish to treat or prevent, and make sure you understand the appropriate therapeutic dosage.

Many health food, nutrition, and specialty stores carry essential oils in small glass bottles at a reasonable price. Many of the oils such as peppermint, orange, or cinnamon are quite inexpensive; you'll pay more for precious flower oils such as rose and jasmine. But because you use essential oils in very tiny quantities, your initial investment is likely to last many years.

Be aware that "perfume" oils are not the same as essential oils. Essential oils are natural plant constituents that have been extracted from the plant. They are oily liquids. Perfume oils are synthetic and are not derived from plants.

THE ETHICS OF HERB-BUYING

Another responsibility you have as an herb consumer is to investigate, when possible, the ethical practices of the supplier. Were the plants cultivated, or were they taken from the wild, a process called "wildcrafting"? If wildcrafted, is the plant plentiful, or is it a rare plant that may be further disrupted by harvesting? Was care taken to avoid harvesting from roadways, under power lines, or near toxic waters or environments? If cultivated, was the plant grown organically? If not, what pesticide or other residues might be in the plant? When was the plant harvested, and how was it processed? Does the grower or harvester process the plant, or was it shipped somewhere else for processing?

CONSULTING AN HERBALIST

You can find an herbalist by checking with the American Herbalist Guild or with the American Association of Naturopathic Physicians. An herbalist or naturopathic physician will want to know all the details about your complaint—how long you've had it, what makes it better or worse, what other complaints might accompany it. Is there an emotional component? Does it interfere with your sleep? Does it change with your diet, the season, your menstrual cycle, the amount of stress you're under? An herbalist will also want to know about your entire state of health, including your medical history—are you healthy otherwise, or do you have other complaints? What do you typically eat and drink? Do you exercise regularly? How do you relax?

In addition to performing a regular physical examination, a naturopathic physician will note the quality of your pulse, the look of your eyes, the glow of your skin, and your general vitality. An herbalist will likely note if you appear tense or sluggish, if you are hot or cold, animated or withdrawn, sharp and alert or dull and out of touch. After spending some time getting to know you, an herbalist can generally make very specific and fine-tuned recommendations.

GATHERING, PREPARING, AND STORING HERBS

Rather than buying herbal remedies or herbs, you can grow and gather the herbs you'd like to use. Harvesting your own herbs and handcrafting them into medicines can be a healing activity in itself!

GATHERING HERBS

Gathering plants you've grown yourself gives you a tremendous sense of accomplishment, but you may also collect herbs growing wild ("wildcrafting"). If you pick wild herbs, however, be certain that you've identified them properly, as some poisonous herbs resemble harmless ones. Take care also that the area in which you're wildcrafting is free of pesticides, chemical sprays, or other pollutants. Avoid picking herbs that grow along busy roads or highways where car exhaust contaminates them. And never harvest rare or endangered plants from the wild.

HARVESTING YOUR HERBS

As a general rule, harvest the leaves of an herb when the plant is about to flower—usually in the spring or fall. Plants are very high in volatile oils right before they flower. Harvest roots and bark in the fall and winter months when the plant is dormant and its nutrients are in storage.

Gather herbs in the morning on a dry day. Herbs that are dry when harvested are less likely to mold or spoil during processing. Avoid washing leaves and flowers of herbs after you've harvested them. If the herbs are covered with dirt or dust, rinse them off with a garden hose or watering can, then allow the herbs to dry for a day or two before picking them. When wildcrafting, shake the water off wet herbs; you may also try drying wild herbs by gently blotting them with a towel. The root of the herb is the only part of the plant that you should wash thoroughly after harvesting.

Harvesting the seeds of an herb requires a little more intuition. You need to check your plants everyday, and be prepared to harvest the seeds as soon as you notice they've begun to dry. Timing is crucial: You must allow the seeds to ripen, but catch them before they fall off the plant. Carefully snap off seed heads over a large paper bag, allowing the seeds to fall into it. Leave the seeds in the bag until they have dried completely.

DRYING HERBS

Herbal preparations often require the use of dried herbs. To dry herbs, hang them upside down until they are crisp. If you have a spare countertop of closet shelf, you can spread the herbs over newspaper or paper towels. Keep the herbs evenly distributed, avoiding thick, wet piles. Cover the herbs with a paper towel or a very thin piece of cheesecloth to prevent dust from settling.

Do not dry herbs in direct sunlight. Dry herbs in an area that is hot, well ventilated, and free of moisture, such as a barn, loft, breezeway, or covered porch. The optimal temperature for drying herbs is approximately 85 degrees Fahrenheit. In these conditions, the moisture will evaporate quickly from the plants, but the aromatic oils will remain in the leaves.

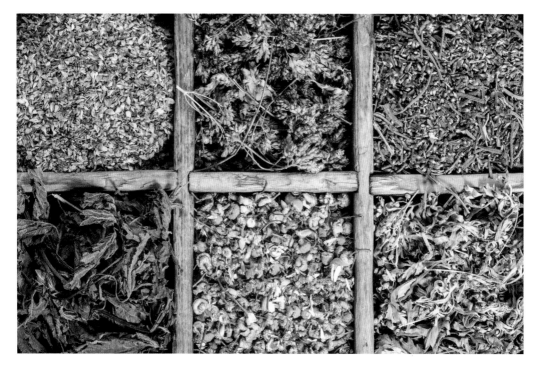

It may take up to a week to dry some herbs, depending on the thickness of the plant's leaves and stem. As soon as leaves are fully dry, but before they become brittle, strip them from the stems. Store the leaves immediately in airtight containers to preserve their flavor and aroma. Label the containers with the herb name and the date stored.

STORING HERBS

Once you've fully dried your herbs, don't delay in storing them in airtight containers or your herbs will lose essential oils, the source of an herb's flavor and perfume.

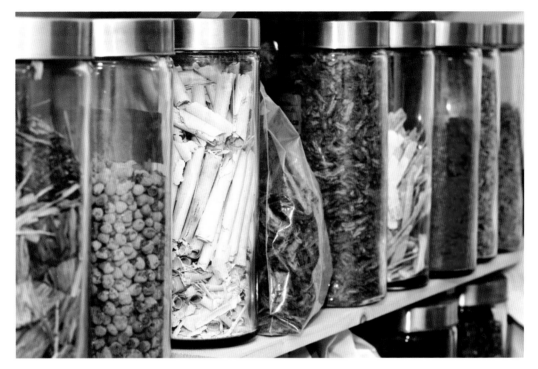

Simply crumble the herbs before storing. Avoid grinding and powdering herbs because they won't retain their flavor as long.

Glass jars with tight-sealing lids or glass stoppers are ideal for storing dried herbs. You may also use porcelain canisters that close tightly, plastic pill holders with tight covers, and sealable plastic bags, buckets, or barrels for large herb pieces.

Store herbs in a dark place to preserve their color and flavor. If you must store herbs in a lighted area, keep them in dark-colored jars that block out most of the light. The worst place to keep herbs in is a spice rack over the stove: Heat from cooking will cause your herbs to lose their flavor quickly. Remember to label each container, including its content and the date of harvest.

MAKING HERBAL MEDICINES

You've grown your herbs, gathered them, and dried them. The next step is to prepare them. Preparing herbs is simple, easy, and economical.

The goal of the herbalist is to release the volatile oils, antibiotics, aromatics, and other healing chemicals an herb contains. You can use dried, powdered herbs to make pills, capsules, and lozenges or add herbs to water to brew infusions, better known as teas. You can soak herbs in alcohol to produce long-lasting tinctures. A spoonful (or more) of sweetener helps the medicine go down in the form of delectable syrups, jellies, and conserves. You can mash herbs for poultices and plasters. Or you can harness the powers of herbs by adding them to make salves, liniments, and creams.

THE FIRST STEPS

Lay out all the cooking, storage, and labeling materials you'll need to prepare your home remedies. Don't attempt to make salves, syrups, and tinctures all at once. Enthusiastic beginners sometimes try to do too much too soon. Even the most experienced practitioner can get confused and make mistakes. Concentrate on making only one type of herbal remedy at a time.

Don't overharvest your herbs. Don't bring in a basketful of rosemary if the recipe calls for no more than an ounce. Think small when you store your herbs, too. Salves and other preparations tend to last longer when stored in small batches. If you intend to save these remedies for longer than a few months, tightly stopper bottles, seal jars with wax, and refrigerate liquid preparations.

Using the basic recipes described in this chapter, you can create your own versions of such delightful herbal preparations as tummy-calming teas, snappy vinegars, and soothing massage oils.

TEAS

One of the easiest and most popular ways of preparing an herbal medicine is to brew a tea. There are two types of teas: infusion and decoctions. If you have ever poured hot water over a tea bag, you have made an infusion, an infusion being herbs steeped in water. A decoction consists of herbs boiled in water. When you simmer cinnamon sticks and cloves in apple cider, you're making a decoction.

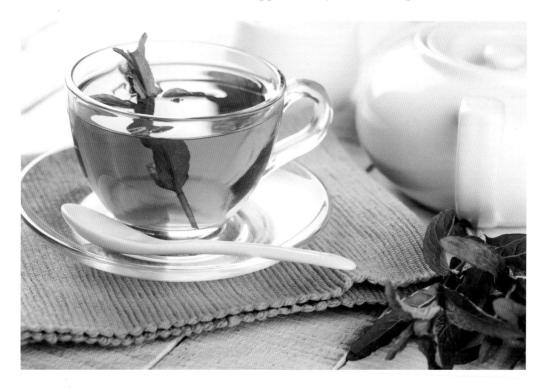

In general, delicate leaves and flowers are best infused, as boiling may cause them to lose the essential oils. To prepare an infusion, use 1 teaspoon of dried herbs per 1 cup of hot water. If you use fresh herbs, use 1 to 2 teaspoons or more. Pour the hot water over the herbs in a pan or teapot, cover with a lid, and allow to steep. You can make your own herbal tea bags, too. Tie up a teaspoon of herbs in a small muslin bag or piece of cheesecloth and drop it in a cup of hot water. Let the tea steep for

15 minutes. To make larger quantities of hot infusions, use 5 tablespoons of herbs per gallon of water.

Roots, barks, and seeds, on the other hand, are best made into decoctions because these hard, woody materials need a bit of boiling to get the constituents out of the fiber. Fresh roots should be sliced thin. To prepare a medicinal decoction use 1 teaspoon of dried herbs per cup of water, cover, and gently boil for 15 to 30 minutes. Use glass, ceramic, or earthenware pots to make your decoction: Aluminum tends to taint herbal teas and impart a bitter taste to them. Strain the decoction. A tea will remain fresh for several days when stored in the refrigerator.

How much of an infusion or decoction can you ingest at one time? In general, drink ½ to 1 cup three times a day. A good rule of thumb is that if you notice no benefits in three days, change the treatment or see your doctor or herbalist. Rely on professional care immediately in case of irregular heartbeat, difficulty breathing, allergic reactions, or severe injuries.

STOMACH REMEDY

1 Tbsp chamomile flowers
1 tsp fennel seeds
2 Tbsp mint leaves

Steep 1 tsp of the mixture in 1 cup of water for 15 minutes; strain and drink.

TINCTURES

Another popular way of making herbal medicines is to produce a tincture. Used for herbs that require a solvent stronger than water to release their chemical constituents, a tincture is an herb extracted in alcohol, glycerine, or vinegar. Tinctures can be added to hot or cold water to make an instant tea or mixed with water for external use in compresses and foot baths. You can even add tinctures to oils or salves to create instant healing ointments. The advantage of tinctures is that they have a long shelf life, and they're available for use in a pinch.

With common kitchen utensils and very little effort, you can easily prepare suitable tinctures. First, clean and pick over fresh herbs, removing any insects or damaged plant material. Remove leaves and flowers from stems and break roots or bark into smaller pieces. Of course, you can use dried herbs, too. Cut or chop the plant parts you want to process or chop in a blender or food processor. Cover with drinking alcohol. The spirits most commonly used are 80 to 100 proof vodka or Everclear. Some herbs, such as ginger and cayenne, require the higher alcohol content to extract their constituents. With other herbs, such as dandelion and nettles, you do not need to use as much alcohol.

Puree the plant material and transfer it to a glass jar. Make sure the alcohol covers the plants. Plant materials exposed to air can mold or rot, so add more alcohol if needed. This is especially important if you use fresh herbs. Store the jar at room temperature out of sunlight, and shake the jar everyday.

After three to six weeks, strain the liquid with a kitchen strainer, cheesecloth, thin piece of muslin, or a paper coffee filter. Even when you've managed to strain out every last bit of plant material, sometimes more particles mysteriously show up after the tincture has been stored. There is no harm in using a tincture that contains a bit of solid debris. Tinctures will keep for many years without refrigeration.

Because the usual dosage of a tincture is 15 to 30 drops, you receive enough herb to benefit from its medicinal properties with very little alcohol. If you don't want to use alcohol for tinctures, you can make vinegar- and glycerine-based tinctures instead. They dissolve plant constituents almost as effectively as spirits.

DANDELION ROOT TINCTURE

Place dried, chopped dandelion roots in a food processor with enough 90 proof vodka to process. Once blended, store in a glass jar, shake daily, and strain in two weeks. Take ½ to 1 tsp three times a day before meals for chronic constipation, poor digestion due to low levels of stomach acid, sick headaches with nausea, or as a spring tonic.

VINEGAR

Vinegar, which contains the solvent acetic acid, is an alternative to alcohol in tinctures—especially for herbs that are high in alkaloids, which require acids to dissolve. You can use herbal vinegars medicinally or dilute them with additional vinegar to make great-tasting salad dressings and marinades.

Use any vinegar with herbs, but to keep your vinegars natural, you may wish to use apple cider vinegar. Apple cider vinegar is made by naturally fermenting apple juice, while white distilled vinegar is an industrial byproduct. Rice vinegar, red wine vinegar, and balsamic vinegar are also good choices, but they are a bit more expensive, and their strong flavors sometimes require additional herbs.

Good herbs for vinegars include basil, cayenne pepper, chives, dill, fennel, garlic, horseradish, marjoram, raspberry, rosemary, tarragon, and thyme.

You can apply a vinegar tincture to the skin to bring down a fever. Dilute the tincture with an equal amount of cool water. Soak a cloth in the solution and bathe the body. As the solution evaporates, it cools the body and therefore lowers the body's temperature. Vinegar is also a potent antifungal agent and makes a good athlete's foot soak when combined with antifungal herbs.

FOOT SOAK VINEGAR

Place two garlic bulbs in a blender along with two handfuls of fresh or dried calendula petals, one handful of chopped fresh comfrey root, and the chopped hulls of several black walnuts (or use ½ oz black walnut tincture). Pour vinegar over the herbs and blend well. Place mixture in a large, shallow pan, and add 20 drops of tea tree oil.

To treat athlete's foot, soak feet in the solution for at least 15 minutes. Rinse feet and dry in the sun or in the light of a sun lamp. Use the foot soak three to four times a day. Make a fresh batch of the mixture for each use.

HERBAL OILS

Oils are a versatile medium for extracting herbal constituents. You may consume herbal oils in recipes or salads, or massage sore body parts with medicinal oils. To make an herbal oil, simply pour oil over herbs and allow the mixture to sit for a week or more.

Olive, almond, canola, sunflower, and sesame are good choices, but any vegetable oil will do. Do not use mineral oil. Strain and bottle. Refrigerate oils you plant to use in cooking.

If you're watching your fat intake, place a good quality herbal oil in a small spray bottle. Before you sauté or stir-fry, spray the pan with a light film of oil. A curried peanut oil or a hot pepper sesame oil adds great taste to a stir-fry. If you need more liquid, add several tablespoons of water.

Good herbs for oils include basil, cayenne pepper, coriander, dill, fennel, garlic, ginger, marjoram, mint, rosemary, tarragon, and thyme.

MASSAGE OIL FOR SORE MUSCLES

5 or 6 cayenne peppers
1 cup vegetable oil
¼ tsp clove essential oil
¼ tsp eucalyptus essential oil
¼ tsp mint essential oil

Chop cayenne peppers and place in a jar. Cover with vegetable oil; make sure the peppers are completely covered. Store oil in a warm, dark place. Strain after one week. Add the essential oils.

Massage on sore muscles. Be careful not to get this oil in your eyes or open wounds, though, as it will sting a lot. Wash your hands after using this oil.

SALVES

Salves, or ointments, are fat-based preparations used to soothe abrasions, heal wounds and lacerations, protect babies' skin from diaper rash, and soften dry, rough skin and chapped lips. Salves are made by heating an herb with fat until the fat absorbs the plant's healing properties. A thickening and hardening agent, such as beeswax, is then added to the strained mixture to give it a thicker consistency.

Kept in a cool place, salves last about six months to a year. You can preserve a salve even longer by adding a few drops of benzoin tincture, poplar bud tincture, or glycerine. (Check pharmacies or health food stores for these items.) Make salves in small batches to keep them fresh. Store in tightly lidded jars.

The key ingredient of salves is herbal oil. Make your oil out of a herb of your choice as described in the previous section. Calendula oil makes a wonderful all-purpose healing salve. Use St. John's wort oil to treat swelling and bruising in traumatic injuries. Use garlic oil in a salve to treat infectious conditions. Good herbs for sore muscles include chamomile, ginger, juniper berries, and lavender. Good herbs to soften and heal skin include aloe vera, calendula, comfrey, marshmallow, and slippery elm.

To turn the oil into a soothing salve, simply mix it with melted beeswax and allow the mixture to become solid. A general rule is to use ¾ to 1 ounce of melted beeswax per 1 cup of herbal oil. Grated beeswax melts faster. Refrigerate the wax before grating to make the job easier. You can melt the beeswax in a double boiler or in a microwave first, or add the grated beeswax to heated herbal oil—it will melt in the warmed oil. Pour the salve into containers before the blend starts to harden.

Note: Problems with your salve? Simply reheat. If you salve is too runny, add a bit more beeswax. If the salve is too hard, use more oil. To test your salve, pour about a tablespoon of salve in a container and put it in the freezer. This "tester" will be ready in a few minutes.

ALL-PURPOSE HEALING SALVE

1 cup comfrey root oil
1 cup calendula oil
2 oz beeswax
2 Tbsp vitamin E oil
20 drops vitamin A emulsion

Grate the beeswax. Combine the oils and gently warm them. Add the beeswax. When the beeswax is melted, add vitamins E and A. Pour into salve containers and let stand to harden.

LINIMENTS

A liniment is a topical preparation that contains alcohol or oil and stimulating, warming herbs such as cayenne. Other warming herbs include eucalyptus, ginger, peppermint, rosemary, and wintergreen. Sometimes isopropyl, or rubbing alcohol, is used instead of grain alcohol. Do not take product made with rubbing alcohol internally. Historically, liniments have been the treatment of choice for aching rheumatic joints and chronic lung congestion.

Liniments warm the skin and turn it red temporarily. It is always a good idea to test your tolerance to a liniment by rubbing a tiny amount on your wrist to make sure it does not burn. To enhance the heat, cover the area with a cloth after application.

LINIMENT FOR ARTHRITIS, LUNG CONGESTION, OR SORE MUSCLES

½ oz cayenne peppers, chopped
½ oz cloves, powdered
1 oz mint leaves
1 oz eucalyptus leaves, chopped
4 cups isopropyl alcohol
60 drops essential oil of wintergreen
20 drops essential oil of peppermint
20 drops essential oil of cloves

Mix all ingredients but essential oils. Store mixture in a dark place at room temperature for two weeks. Strain or press out fluids. Add essential oils and stir well. Massage liniment into arthritic joints, sore muscles, or onto back and chest for congestion.

CREAMS

A cream differs from a salve or a liniment in that its liquid portion blends together with the oil. Because creams often contain water or other liquids, they are less greasy than salves and liniments. Making a cream is like making mayonnaise or gravy. Slowly add liquid to the warm wax and oil solution until the ingredients combine smoothly.

CALENDULA-LAVENDER CREAM

½ tsp hydrous lanolin (available in pharmacies)
½ oz beeswax, grated
2 oz comfrey oil
2 oz calendula oil
2 oz calendula succus (fresh juice preserved with a bit of alcohol)
$^1/_{16}$ oz borax powder
¼ tsp lavender essential oil

Mix and heat oils. Melt lanolin and beeswax in the warmed oils. In another pot, gently warm succus and dissolve borax in it. Remove both mixtures from heat. Add succus to first mixture very slowly, while constantly whisking. Stir in lavender oil. Spoon into jars and seal. Cream made from fresh plant juices tends to go bad after 6 to 12 months. Store in the refrigerator.

LOTIONS

When you mix an herbal tincture or tea such as slippery elm or comfrey with an oil, it forms a thin, soothing liquid. Add essential oils for therapeutic purposes or just to create a scented lotion.

SOOTHING LOTION

1 oz calendula tincture
1½ oz comfrey tincture
½ oz vitamin E oil
1 oz aloe vera gel or fresh pulp
¼ tsp vitamin C crystals
essential oil, if desired

Pour ingredients into a bottle and shake vigorously.

COMPRESSES AND POULTICES

You can use compresses to treat headaches, sore muscles, itching, and swollen glands, among other conditions. To make a compress, soak a cloth in a strong herbal tea, wring it out, and place it on the skin.

Soak a cloth with strong peppermint tea to treat rashes that itch and burn. Soak a cloth in cayenne powder tea to apply to an aching arthritic joint. Or soak a cloth with St. John's wort or arnica tincture and hold against a sprained ankle.

Good herbs for compresses include garlic, ginger, marjoram, sage, St. John's wort, and witch hazel.

To make a poultice, mash herbs with enough water to form a paste. Place the herb match directly on the affected boy part and cover with a clean white cloth or gauze.

Good herbs for poultices include comfrey, marshmallow, mustard, oatmeal, and slippery elm bark.

MUSTARD PLASTER

A mustard poultice is a time-honored therapy: Your great-grandmother may have used mustard poultices and plasters to treat congestion, coughs, bronchitis, or pneumonia. A mustard plaster offers immediate relief to chest discomfort and actually helps to treat infectious conditions—a much-needed remedy in the days before antibiotics. It works mainly by increasing circulation, perspiration, and heat in the afflicted area

The best poultices are made from black mustard seeds ground fresh in a coffee grinder, but ordinary yellow mustard will do in a pinch.

To prepare a mustard poultice, mix ½ cup mustard powder with 1 cup flour. Stir hot water into the mustard and flour mixture until it forms a paste. Spread the mixture on a piece of cotton or muslin that has been soaked in hot water. Cover with a second piece of dry material.

The person receiving the treatment should sit or lie down comfortably. Lay the moist side of the poultice across the person's chest or back. A second poultice can be placed on the back if desired.

Leave the poultice on for 15 to 30 minutes; promptly remove if the person experiences any discomfort. The procedure is likely to promote perspiration and reddening of the chest. Give the individual plenty of liquids during the procedure and encourage her to take a warm or cool shower afterward, then rest or gently stretch for a half hour.

HERBAL BATHS

Add healing herbs to bath or foot soaks; the skin absorbs the properties of many herbs. Any herb that you can use to make a tea, you can also use to make a bath or foot soak. Just add a pint of herbal infusion or a decoction to the water. You can also try placing herbs in a muslin bag and then suspending the bag under the hot water tap.

All-purpose herbs for baths include lavender, lemon balm, and rosemary. Herbs that boost circulation include ginger, lavender, rosemary, and yarrow. Herbs for restful sleep include chamomile, hops, lavender, and valerian.

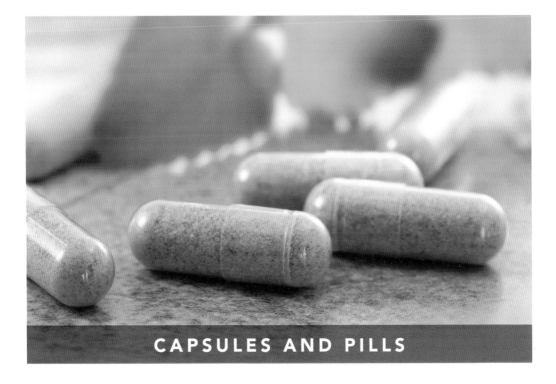

CAPSULES AND PILLS

You can buy herbal capsules, tablets, and lozenges at a natural food store or make your own. Capsules and tablets provide a convenient method of ingesting herbs that have strong, harsh flavors. People who do not enjoy drinking herbal teas or using alcohol-based tinctures may also prefer taking herbs in pill form.

You can purchase empty gelatin capsules at health food stores and at some pharmacies, or by ordering them online. When making encapsulated herbs fill one half of the capsule with the powdered herb and pack tightly. (A chopstick works well to pack the powdered herbs into the capsule.) Close with the other half of the capsule. It takes only a couple of minutes to make a week's supply of herbal capsules.

To make pills, blend powdered herbs with a bit of honey to bind the mixture. Pinch off bits of the resulting sticky substance and roll into balls. If the balls seems too moist, roll them in a mixture of slippery elm and licorice powder to soak up the extra moisture. Dry the herbal pills in a dehydrator, an oven set to preheat, or outdoors on a warm day covered with a cloth. Store the dried pills in an airtight container.

Note that it's best to store your herbs whole or crumbled in large pieces. Don't powder them until immediately before encapsulating them. Use a mortar or pestle. For harder roots, barks, or seeds, try powdering them in a coffee grinder or food processor.

RELAXATION PILLS

Combine equal parts of powdered skullcap, valerian, rosemary, chamomile, and peppermint. Blend with honey to bind. Roll off pill-sized pieces, dry, and store in a tightly sealed container. Use to relieve tension and calm anxiety.

LOZENGES

To make herbal lozenges, combine powdered herbs with sugar and a mucilaginous binding agent such as marshmallow root, licorice root*, or slippery elm bark.

THROAT LOZENGES

3 Tbsp licorice powder*
3 Tbsp slippery elm powder
1 Tbsp myrrh powder

1 tsp cayenne powder
honey as needed
20 drops orange essential oil
2 drops thyme essential oil

Mix herbal powders. Stir in honey until a gooey mass forms. Add essential oils and mix very well. Spread the paste on a marble slab or other nonstick surface coated with sugar or cornstarch. With a rolling pin, roll the mixture flat to about the thickness of a pancake.

Sprinkle with sugar and cornstarch. With a knife, cut into small, separate squares. Or pinch off pieces and roll into ¼-inch balls. Flatten the balls into round lozenges and let dry. Allow lozenges to air-dry in a well-ventilated area for 12 hours. Suck on lozenges to help heal sore throats or coughs.

*Do not use licorice if you have high blood pressure.

SYRUPS

Even the most bitter herbs can taste good when made into syrups. Syrups are ideal for soothing sore throats and respiratory ailments. You can make herbal syrups by mixing sugar, honey, or glycerine with infusions, decoctions, tinctures, herbal juices, or medicinal liquors. (Refined sugar makes a clearer syrup with a better flavor.)

To preserve syrup, refrigerate or make them with glycerine. Glycerine both sweetens and preserves the mixture. Alcohol may also be added, but syrups made with glycerine are better for children.

Make syrups in small quantities. To make a simple syrup, dissolve the sweetener of your choice in a hot herb infusion. You can add herbal tinctures to increase the

syrup's medicinal value. (Add 1 to 2 ounces of tincture to the formula on this page, if you wish.) Strain, if necessary, and bottle. Keep refrigerated.

HERBAL SYRUP

¼ cup sugar or honey
½ cup glycerine
1½ cups strong herb infusion

Combine sweetener and infusion in a pan and bring to a boil. Add glycerine. Pour into clean bottles and let cool. Keep refrigerated. Makes about 2 cups of syrups.

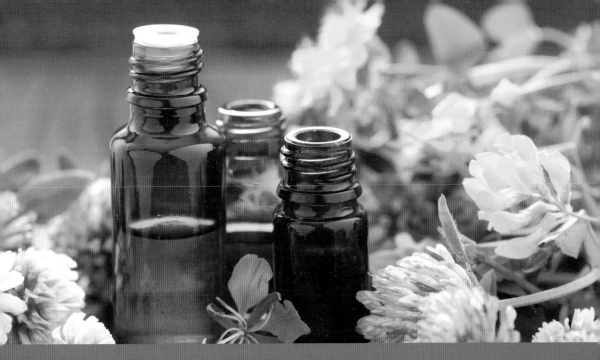

AROMATHERAPY

Aroma means scent, and therapy means treatment. Aromatherapy, then, is the use of the fragrant parts of aromatic plants to improve your health and general well being. First, of course, aromatherapy offers pure enjoyment. Taking a whiff of a spice in your kitchen or a bouquet of flowers is fundamental aromatherapy.

Aromatherapy has many other benefits, too. Inhaling the appropriate fragrance can reduce stress, lift a depression, hasten a good night's sleep, soothe your soul, or give you more energy. Massaging aromatic oils into your skin is another way to benefit from aromatherapy. That's because essential oils, the compounds responsible for a plant's fragrance, offer a multitude of healing benefits in addition to their individual scents. A pungent liniment such as Chinese Tiger Balm, for instance, eases aches and pains. And the latest fragrant shampoos and body oils will improve the health of your complexion and hair while at the same time inducing a particular mood. Aromatherapy, then, is very versatile and can be used in many different ways to treat a wide range of physical and emotional problems.

SCENT IN HISTORY

The burning of fragrant woods, leaves, needles, and tree gums as incense is thought to be the earliest form of aromatherapy. This practice probably arose from the discovery that some firewoods, such as cypress and cedar, filled the air with scent when they burned. In fact, our modern word perfume is derived from the Latin *per fumum*, which means "through smoke."

Incense was not the only early use of fragrance, however. Sometime between 7000 and 4000 B.C. Neolithic tribes learned that animal fats, when heated, absorbed plants' aromatic and healing properties. Perhaps fragrant leaves or flowers accidentally dropped into fat as meat cooked over the fire. The information gleaned from that accident led to other discoveries: Such plants added flavor to food, helped heal wounds, and smoothed dry skin far better than nonscented fat. These fragrant fats, the forerunners of our modern massage and body lotions, scented the wearer, protected skin and hair from weather and insects, and relaxed aching muscles. They also affected people's energies and emotions.

Aromatic water, a third type of fragrant product, was actually a combination of essential oils, water, and alcohol. It was used to enhance the complexion and scent the skin and hair. It also was ingested as a medicinal tonic. It was the forerunner of our modern perfume.

As civilization became more advanced, incense, body oils, and aromatic waters were combined into blends to heal the mind, body, and spirit. Thus, throughout the world, aroma became an integral part of healing and lay the foundation for our use of aromatherapy today.

BABYLONIAN BEGINNINGS

Today, cities prosper and fail with the price of oil. So, too, did they in ancient times; however, it was fragrant oils and spices, not fuel oil, that sparked the growth of key cities along the avenues of commerce. No one knows exactly when trade began, but an import order for cedarwood, myrrh, and cypress was found inscribed on an early Babylonian clay tablet. More than 5,000 years ago, when Egyptians were just learning to write and make bricks, they were already bringing in large quantities of myrrh—their most valued trade import. Certainly there were trade routes through the Middle East to obtain myrrh and other fragrant goods before 2000 B.C., and these routes were well-traveled for the next 30 centuries.

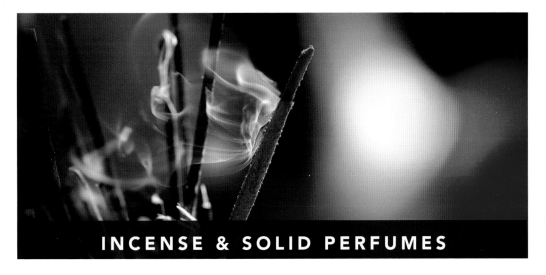

INCENSE & SOLID PERFUMES

For thousands of years and throughout the world, fragrant smoke has purified the air and comforted individuals who were in physical, emotional, or spiritual need. At first, tossing a few fragrant plant twigs into the fire served the purpose, but eventually solid incense was created using ground gums and plants mixed with honey. These were formed into solid cubes and set on a coal from the fire. In many cultures, elaborate ceremonial burners were designed to hold cubes of incense atop smoldering coals. The ancients filled temples, council rooms, and homes with incense, using it even more liberally than we would an air freshener. Small wonder, since incense was able to dispel the disagreeable smells of unsanitary living conditions.

In Europe, Arabia, India, China, and throughout North America, dwellings were fumigated to drive out the evil spirits that were believed to cause illness while, at the same time, ridding the dwelling of fleas and bugs. During epidemics, people who flocked to temples and churches were probably helped by the burning of antiseptic herbs. Hippocrates, the father of medicine, is said to have freed Athens from the plague by burning aromatic plants, as did Moses and Aaron in the desert.

Respiratory and rheumatic ills, headaches, unconsciousness, and other medical problems were treated by breathing in smoke arising from aromatic plants. And sometimes wet, aromatic herbs or herb teas were dropped on hot rocks to create a steam that was inhaled. Both techniques proved effective in treating sinus congestion, lung problems, or earache.

During religious and healing ceremonies, Native Americans burned tight bundles of fragrant herbs and braids of the vanillalike sweet grass and surrounded themselves in the smoke. And to heal the sick, rocks steaming from the tea of goldenrod, fleabane, pearly everlasting, and echinacea were placed next to a patient, and both were covered with hides or blankets to make a type of aroma-filled mini-sauna.

Throughout Europe, Arabia, and India, incense proved to be immensely versatile; it was used as perfume, medicine, and even mouthwash. Remember, early incense contained nothing other than ground herbs, plant gums, and honey. (Only much later was messy charcoal and inedible saltpeter added so that, once ignited, it would continue burning.) Since most of the herbs were highly antiseptic, when rubbed on the skin and melted by body heat, they released a scent and disinfected wounds. Incense was even ingested as medicine. It is no surprise, then, that the Greek word *arómata* had several meanings: incense, perfume, spice, and aromatic medicine. The Chinese also had one word, *heang,* to describe perfume, incense, and the concept of fragrance.

Some aromatics were even found to help with weight loss, digestion, or menstrual regularity. Rome's most famous perfume, Susinon, when ingested was a diuretic and relieved various types of inflammation. Amarakinon treated indigestion and hemorrhoids and encouraged menstruation, either when ingested or applied directly to the affliction. It was also worn as perfume. Spikenard was the main ingredient in another perfume that could be sucked as a throat lozenge to relieve coughs and laryngitis.

Throughout the world, incense has been employed to affect mind and emotions. According to the Japanese, it fosters communication with the transcendent, purifies mind and body, keeps you alert, acts as a companion in the midst of solitude, and brings moments of peace amidst busy affairs. The fragrant smoke billowing from Chinese bronze incense burners was classified into six basic moods: tranquil, reclusive, luxurious, beautiful, refined, and noble.

BODY OILS THROUGH HISTORY

Fragrance also found its way into religious and secular life via scented oils. These were made, as they still are today, by extracting plant oils into fat or vegetable oil and then straining out the used plant material. They were used liberally in religious ceremonies to consecrate temples, alters, statues, candles, and priests. The Book of Exodus (30:22-25), for example, provides one of the earliest recipes for an anointing oil—given by God to Moses to be used in the initiation of priests. The ingredients included myrrh, cinnamon, calamus, and cassia blended into olive oil.

Egyptian talent for formulating scented oils became legendary, and their oils were certainly potent: Calcite pots filled with richly scented oils still held a faint odor when King Tutankamen's tomb was opened 3,000 years later. Egyptians were especially creative with the use of scent and did not restrict it to religious rites. An individual's special odor, or khaibt, was represented by a hieroglyph of a fan and was thought capable of influencing the emotions of others.

THE FIRST BEAUTY SPA?

The first beauty spa may have been the perfume factory owned by Cleopatra at En Gedi, by the Dead Sea. Individuals were apparently offered health and beauty treatments, since the ruins of the factory show seats in what are believed to have been waiting and treatment rooms. Fragrant herbs were blended into specially prepared olive oil. Unfortunately, the book in which Cleopatra recorded recipes for her body oils, *Cleopatra Gynaeciarum Libri,* is long lost. We know of it only through its mention in Roman texts.

The Romans, who did not enjoy the messy process of infusing and straining scented oils, imported most of theirs from Egypt. Men and women alike literally bathed in fragrance. So prevalent was the use of scent that Romans affectionately called their sweethearts "my myrrh, my cinnamon," just as today we call our loved ones "honey."

The Greeks were especially attracted to the use of scented oils. In fact, Hippocrates recommended the use of body oils in the bath. In Athens, proprietors of unguentarii shops sold marjoram, lily, thyme, sage, anise, rose, and iris infused in oil and thickened with beeswax. They packaged their unguents (from a word meaning to smear or anoint) in small, elaborately decorated ceramic pots, as they still do today.

However, in those times the shopkeepers were consulted as doctors, and their products were sold for a multitude of medicinal uses.

The daily bathing ritual in India required the application of sesame oils scented with jasmine, coriander, cardamom, basil, costus, pandanus, agarwood, pine, saffron, champac, and clove. Ancient Vedic religious and medical books gave instruction on balancing body temperature, temperament, and digestion with such aromas, and some of their therapeutic uses were certainly passed on to the West.

In Egypt, everyone used body oils, from royalty to laborers. Builders constructing a burial site went on strike in the twelfth century B.C. not just because the food was bad, but even worse, they complained, "We have no ointment." They depended upon the oils to ease sore muscles after a day of hauling and carving huge stones and to protect their skin from the intense Egyptian sun.

Throughout the Americas, massage with scented oils was also used as therapy and was often the first treatment given. One massage oil prepared by the Incas contained valerian and other relaxing herbs that were thickened with seaweed. The Aztecs massaged the sick with scented ointments in their sweat lodges.

THE HISTORY OF PERFUME

Perfume as we know it today—packaged in tiny, expensive bottles with a high alcohol content and hundreds of chemical compounds—is a relatively new invention. The first written description of a distiller to produce essential oils appears around the first century A.D. Maria Prophetissa, known as Mary the Jewess, invented a mechanism that looked something like a double-boiler. She described the essential oil it produced as an "angel who descends from the sky." By the second century A.D. the Chinese and Arabs were distilling essential oils, and Japan followed suit a few centuries later.

CHEMISTRY AND COSMETICS

A little more than 100 years ago, the fragrance industry was suddenly thrust into the modern chemical age. Previously, cologne and even soap had always been considered part of the medicinal pharmacy. Then, in 1867, the Paris International Exhibition boldly exhibited them in a separate section dubbed cosmetics. This radical move birthed an entirely new industry that paved the way for a new product: perfume.

The very next year, the first commercial synthetic essential oil was developed in the laboratory. With its fresh smell of newly mowed hay, the synthetic oil was an instant hit with cologne manufacturers. Thousands of synthetic fragrances, even those imitating the rarest and most expensive essential oils, were engineered mostly from petroleum chemicals.

These synthetic oils changed the character of personal fragrance forever. The new chemicals were so concentrated, they allowed the manufacture of powerful perfumes. Replacing light colognes that were liberally splashed on, just a few small drops of perfume completely scented an individual. Still other newly-invented chemical additives made that scent linger for hours. Of course, with all the synthetic ingredients, colognes and perfumes were no longer medicinal—and certainly not edible. For the first time in history, they were purely a cosmetic product.

AROMATHERAPY COMES OF AGE

Today, perfume, food, medicine, and aromatherapy products are viewed as separate entities, although aromatherapy is slowly reclaiming its medicinal heritage. A French chemist, René-Maurice Gattefossé, coined the term *aromatherapie* in 1928. His family were perfumers, but his interest in the therapeutic use of essential oils began when he severely burned his hand in a laboratory explosion. He deliberately plunged his hand into a nearby container of lavender oil to ease the pain, but was amazed at how quickly it healed. He wrote numerous books and papers on the chemistry of perfume and cosmetics. Around the same time another Frenchman, Albert Couvreur, published a book on the medicinal uses of essential oils.

A new wave of aromatherapist practitioners was inspired by this work, one of whom was Dr. Jean Valnet, who, while an army surgeon during World War II, used essential oils such as thyme, clove, lemon, and chamomile on wounds and burns. He later used essential oils to treat psychiatric problems. Marguerite Maury, a French biochemist, developed therapeutic methods for applying these oils to the skin as a massage, reintroducing an ancient method of aromatherapy to the modern world.

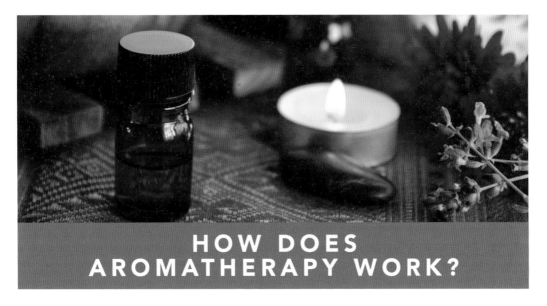

HOW DOES AROMATHERAPY WORK?

Remember the heady fragrance of an herb or flower garden on a hot summer's day, or the crisp smell of an orange as you peel it? These odors are the fragrance of the plant's essential oils, the potent, volatile, and aromatic substance contained in various parts of the plant, including its flowers, leaves, roots, wood, seeds, fruit, and bark. The essential oils carry concentrations of the plant's healing properties—those same properties that traditional Western medicine utilizes in many drugs. Professional aromatherapists focus very specifically on the controlled use of essential oils to treat ailments and disease and to promote physical and emotional well-being.

Aromatherapy doesn't just work through the sense of smell alone, however. Inhalation is only one application method. Essential oils can also be applied to the skin. When used topically, the oils penetrate the skin, taking direct action on body tissues and organs in the vicinity of application. They also enter the bloodstream and are carried throughout the body. Of course, when applied topically the fragrance of the essential oil is also inhaled.

There are three different modes of action in the body: pharmacological, which affects the chemistry of the body; physiological, which affects the ability of the body to function and process; and psychological, which affects emotions and attitudes. These three modes interact continuously. Aromatherapy is so powerful partly because it affects all three modes. You choose the application method based on where you most want the effects concentrated and on what is most convenient and pleasing to you.

Aromatherapy is actually an aspect of herbal medicine. Herbal medicine also utilizes the healing powers of plants to treat physical and emotional problems, but it uses the whole plant or parts of the plant, such as leaves, flowers, roots, and seeds, rather than the essential oil. Aromatherapy and herbal medicine can be used individually, or they can be used jointly to augment potential healing benefits.

THERAPEUTIC USES OF ESSENTIAL OILS

You can treat a wide range of physical problems with aromatherapy. Almost all essential oils have antiseptic properties and are able to fight infection and destroy bacteria, fungi, yeast, parasites, and/or viruses. Many essential oils also reduce aches and pain, soothe or rout inflammations and spasms, stimulate the immune system and insulin and hormone production, affect blood circulation, dissolve mucus and open nasal passages, or aid digestion—just to mention a few of their amazing properties.

Aromatherapy can also have a considerable influence on our emotions. Sniffing clary sage, for example, can quell panic, while the fragrance released by peeling an orange can make you feel more optimistic. Since your mind strongly influences your health and is itself a powerful healing tool, it makes aromatherapy's potential even more exciting.

Many essential oils perform more than one function, so having just a half-dozen or so on hand will help you treat a wide range of common physical ailments and emotional problems.

The beauty of aromatherapy is that you can create a blend of oils that will benefit both in one treatment. For example, you can blend a combination of essential oils that not only stops indigestion, but also reduces the nervous condition that encouraged it. Or, you could design an aromatherapy body lotion that both improves your complexion and relieves depression.

THE ESSENCE OF ESSENTIAL OILS

Plants take the light of the sun, the minerals of the earth, and the carbon dioxide exhaled by humans and animals and, through photosynthesis, transform them into the building blocks of medicine. Among the most important therapeutic compounds manufactured by plants are essential oils. These volatile oils contain a variety of active constituents and are also responsible for each plant's unique fragrance.

The basic elements of carbon, hydrogen, and oxygen combine to form the different organic molecular compounds that produce aromas. So far, more than 30,000 of

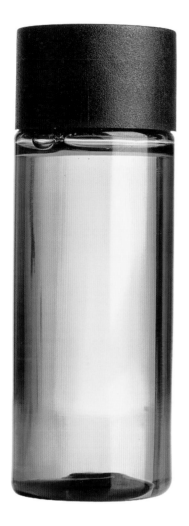

these molecular compounds have been identified and named. Most individual essential oils consist of many different aromatic molecular compounds. In fact, the essential oil from just one plant may contain as many as one hundred different fragrance molecules. In nature there are thousands of plants, all with unique fragrances that are comprised of different combinations of these molecules.

Plants that smell similar to one another usually contain some of the same molecular compounds. Lemon verbena, lemon balm (melissa), lemon thyme, lemon eucalyptus, citronella, lemongrass, and lemon itself, for instance, all smell like lemon because they contain a lemon-scented molecule called citral. But it is the other aromatic molecules they contain that give each plant its unique fragrance.

Aromatic compounds are grouped under larger classes of compounds. Each molecular compound has characteristic scents and actions on the body. Some may be cooling and relaxing, while others are warming and stimulating. Some are better for treating indigestion, while others are antiseptic.

Every effect of an essential oil has a chemical explanation. These effects include their biological activity in the body (beneficial, irritating, or toxic), their solubility (in oil or alcohol, for instance), how rapidly they evaporate in air or are absorbed through the skin, and how well different oils combine as scents.

The proportion of aromatic compounds in a particular type of plant is not necessarily constant. This proportion can change from year to year depending on the plant's growing conditions, including geographic location, elevation, climate, soil quality, and the methods used to harvest it and extract the essential oil.

THE PHYSIOLOGY OF SCENT

Essential oil molecules enter the body through the nose and the skin. Since these molecules are extremely small and float easily through the air, you can simply inhale them into your lungs, which then disperse them into your bloodstream. The blood quickly carries them throughout your body. Essential oil molecules are also small enough to be absorbed through the pores of the skin. Once absorbed, some molecules enter the bloodstream, while others remain in the area of application or evaporate into the air. How much goes where depends on the size of the essential oil molecules, the method of application (massage increases absorption), and the carrier containing the essential oil, be it alcohol, vegetable oil, vinegar, or water. This makes essential oils perfect for healing a specific skin problem as well as the entire body.

The sense of smell has its own important mechanisms. High in the nose is the olfactory epithelium, two smell receptors about the size of dimes. The receptors pick up volatile and lipid-soluble molecules using tiny filaments called cilia, which may actually be able to identify odor molecules by their "shape." It is believed that these odor receptors are coded by a huge family of genes to sense particular components of smell that produce a characteristic "fingerprint" pattern of activity in the brain.

From the olfactory mucus membrane, signals travel to olfactory bulbs that extend forward like tiny spoons from the brain. An electrical impulse then goes directly to the limbic system, which is part of what is called the primitive or "old" brain.

Smell, it seems, was our first sense, and our old brain actually evolved from the olfactory stalks. Because recognition of smell moves directly into the old brain, it completely bypasses areas that control reasoning and the central nervous system. Thus, it directly influences survival mechanisms such as "fight or flight" reactions and the autonomic functions of the body, including heartbeat, body temperature, appetite, digestion, sexual arousal, and memory—the functions we can't control by will or reason. It also affects instincts such as emotions, attraction/repulsion, lust, and creativity. The senses of hearing and vision, by contrast, first stimulate the thalamus, which registers only warmth and pain. Furthermore, the old brain is directly connected to the hypothalamus and pituitary glands, and therefore to our immune system and hormones, which is why smell affects them so powerfully.

ESSENTIAL OILS AND OUR DAILY LIVES

Have you ever smelled a certain flower or cologne and suddenly experienced déjà vu? Or perhaps you've caught a whiff of fir and immediately envisioned a Christmas tree even in the middle of July. Scent can transport us back to previous experiences, triggering long forgotten feelings associated with those memories. That's because a particular aroma triggers areas of the brain that influence your emotions, memory, cardiovascular functioning, and hormonal balance. Your body thinks you are there!

In fact, memories associated with scent influence us more than most of us realize. Realtors know that the smell of baking cookies, heightened by the aroma of vanilla, can sell a house because it reminds potential buyers of being nurtured. In fact, realtors can forgo the cookies and simply scent the air with a vanilla fragrance.

Memory and association are only one way scents affect us psychologically. According to researchers studying aromacology, the science of medicinal aromas, fragrance actually alters our brain waves.

For instance, stimulating scents such as peppermint and eucalyptus intensify brain waves, making the mind sharper and clearer. The effects are similar to those of coffee, but are achieved without caffeine's detrimental impact on the adrenal glands. As a result, aroma can help workers such as truck drivers and air traffic controllers, whose jobs—and the safety of others—depend on their being attentive.

Certain fragrances can also produce the opposite effect. If you inhale a flowery draft of chamomile tea, your brain waves will lengthen, causing you to feel relaxed. This is similar to the effect of taking a sedative drug but without the concomitant liver damage.

Some essential oils have effects similar to antidepressant drugs, according to the Olfaction Research Group at Warwick University in England. Italian psychiatrist Paolo Rovesti, M.D., helped is patients overcome depression using the scents of various citruses, such as orange, bergamot, lemon, and lemon verbena.

Psychologists help people overcome anxiety, tension, and mood swings by having them associate a scent with feelings of rest and contentment. The psychologist uses biofeedback or visualization techniques to help the client relax, and then sniff a relaxing scent. Later, the client can simply smell the relaxation scent when he or she becomes nervous or anxious.

PURCHASING ESSENTIAL OILS

In order to be an educated consumer and purchase good quality essential oils for aromatherapy, you need to understand how an essential oil is extracted from the plant as well as what differentiates a good quality essential oil from a poor quality one. You can't tell just by looking. But using a high quality oil is essential to achieving maximum healing benefits from your aromatherapy treatments. And, in the long run, buying high quality oils will be easier on your pocketbook, too.

HOW ESSENTIAL OILS ARE PRODUCED

There are several different ways to extract essential oils, and all require elaborate equipment. As you will see from the following descriptions, most extraction techniques are based on the fact that the majority of essential oils mix with oils, fats, alcohol, and certain solvents, but not with water. Some methods are more suitable for certain plants than others, depending on the plant's chemical make-up.

DISTILLATION

Most pure essential oils are extracted from plants through steam distillation. Freshly picked plants are suspended over boiling water, and the steam pulls the oils out of the plant. The steam rises, is captured in a vessel, and is pushed along tubing. Then the steam is rapidly cooled, causing it to condense back into water. Since water and essential oils do not mix, the two separate, and the essential oil is collected.

A byproduct of this distillation is the remaining water. Some plants contain aromatic compounds that are so water soluble, they remain in the water that is left over after distillation. Such waters are very fragrant and are prized by aromatherapists, who refer to them as hydrosols. In aromatherapy, hydrosols are used mostly in cosmetics to moisturize skin.

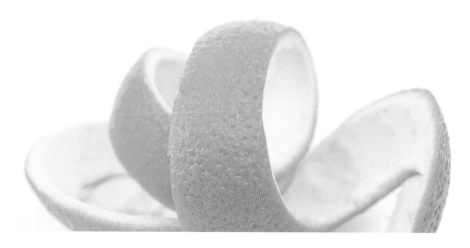

EXPRESSION

The most direct method of producing essential oils is pressing them from the plant's flesh, seeds, and skins, a process similar to that used to obtain olive oil. This technique is used mostly with citrus peels, such as orange, lemon, lime, or grapefruit, because the oil in their peels is easily pressed out.

ENFLEURAGE

This very old method is rarely used today except in France. It is a long and complicated process that has become very expensive. Blossoms are set on sheets of warm fat that absorb the oil from the flowers. Originally animal fat or lard was used, but now vegetable fats are more common. Once the essential oil has been incorporated into the fat, the "exhausted" flowers are removed and replaced with fresh ones. The process is repeated several times until the fat is infused with fragrance. Then the fat is separated out with solvents, leaving just the essential oil.

SOLVENTS

Aromatherapists tend to shy away from oils obtained through chemical solvents, worrying that slight traces of the solvent may remain even though they are supposed to be completely removed. First, the plant is dissolved in a solvent such as benzene, hexane, or chlorure of methylene. The solvent, which has a low boiling point, is then evaporated off, sometimes with the help of a machine that uses vacuum or centrifugal force to help pull it away from the essential oil. The resulting oils are called "absolutes." A similar method uses paraffin waxes as the solvent, but does not evaporate them off. Instead, the remaining paraffins cause the final product to be solid, and thus it is called "concrete."

Even though the evaporated solvent is recaptured and cooled back into liquid so that it can be reused, this process is still expensive. As a result, it is reserved for costly oils that cannot be distilled, such as jasmine and vanilla, or for rose essential oil, which is slightly less expensive when obtained through this process rather than through distillation.

QUALITY

Since they are products of nature, the quality of essential oils is affected by growing conditions, the particular species of plant, extraction techniques, and storage, among other factors. Even the type of soil, temperature, and cloud cover affect some oils. To determine the quality of an essential oil, you'll need to be concerned with three crucial characteristics: purity, grade, and integrity. The information below and lots of experience will guide you.

PURITY

Purity is an important concern to anyone purchasing essential oils. They can be adulterated, cut, or entirely replaced with a cheaper substitute or extended or diluted with vegetable oils, alcohol, or solvents. These substitutes and extenders might not be derived from a plant at all. But even if they are, the oil will not be as potent as it should be, nor will it function as expected. Unfortunately, a label claiming a product is a pure essential oil is no guarantee that it is the real thing. An oil labelled rose or vanilla may have been produced in a laboratory out of synthetic chemicals, but it can still be labeled an essential oil.

Inexpensive oils such as orange, cedar, or peppermint are seldom altered. However, alteration is common with expensive oils that are in great demand, such as rose, melissa, and jasmine.

Dilution with vegetable oil is usually easy to detect. Dilution with alcohol may be a bit more difficult to determine, but these oils do have a slight alcohol odor. Oils adulterated with a clear, non-oily solvent are the most difficult to recognize. This is a potential health hazard as well, since such solvents are readily absorbed into the body when rubbed on the skin or inhaled through the lungs.

GRADES

Many essential oils are sold to distributors in different grades. Their prices often reflect this: The better grades command up to double the cost of the lesser grades. For example, lavender is commonly available in at least a dozen different grades and lemon in four. The lesser grades are often still pure essential oil, but they contain less of the most important aromatic principles.

Different processing methods can produce different grades. For example, redistillation produces oil that is stronger in some compounds than others. This is typically done with peppermint oil so the chewing gum and candy it flavors has a lighter, fresher taste and smell.

Once your nose has had a little experience with essential oils, you'll find that higher grades generally are more intense and carry a richer bouquet of fragrance.

Lower quality oils usually smell less complicated or weak because they do not contain a full range of aromatic compounds.

When two bottles of the same kind of oil smell differently, it does not necessarily mean that one is better than the other. The best quality oils are similar to fine wine in that even experts don't agree on their favorites. For example, one geranium essential oil might carry a distinctly stronger hint of citrus while another smells more like rose. Which is better? Most people will prefer the rose, but that doesn't make it better.

INTEGRITY

By integrity we mean that the oil is pure and natural and comes from a single species of plant (and probably even from the same region and harvest). An oil with integrity is not whipped up in a laboratory or composed of cheaper essential oils. But inexpensive lemongrass or citronella essential oils sometimes masquerade as the very expensive melissa (lemon balm) oil. To make an artificial rose oil in the laboratory, rose geranium may be used as a starting point, then chemically altered to mimic, although never completely accurately, a rose scent.

The problem here is that although the end product still contains only pure, natural essential oils, it will not have the properties you want and expect. Asking for an oil by its Latin name may help, but it doesn't guarantee that you will get what you want.

SHOPPING FOR ESSENTIAL OILS

At first, it may seem a formidable task to detect the difference between good and poor grades of oil or to spot a synthetic. But you'll be pleasantly surprised at how easy it becomes, after only a little practice, to sniff out good essential oils.

Until your nose knows, you'll have to trust your source. Each essential oil company decides the quality it will offer. Some companies consistently sell the poorer, cheaper grades while others prefer to sell the higher grades. They will rarely offer you, as a retail consumer, a choice in grades. As a result, some lines tend to be more expensive than others. But do not use price alone to judge an oil's quality, since lower grades of oil may be sold for far more than they are worth. Remember, too, that store clerks do not always know much about aromatherapy and may naively think that anything labeled an essential oil comes from the plant named.

Sophisticated advertising and fancy packaging may also be misleading. And, because not everyone cares about the healing effects, a few companies have filled the growing demand for scents with the cheapest means at their disposal. The most unscrupulous will sell low quality oils for the price of better ones.

This being said, you will find oils and related supplies at natural food stores, herb stores, specialty mail-order catalogs, and of course, at aromatherapy and skin care outlets. Some stores also have retail sites on the Internet. Some essential oil mail-order companies are run by aromatherapists who stake their reputation on supplying high quality oils, so they may be the best way for you to get what you want. However, you need to know exactly what you want since you will not have the opportunity to sniff before purchase.

PRICE

There is great variation in the price of essential oils because some are more expensive to produce. For instance, rose oil is expensive because the flowers must be carefully cultivated, pruned, and hand-picked. Jasmine oil is expensive for similar reasons. Producing an ounce of pure jasmine requires 20 days labor for an experienced picker, followed by costly methods of extraction. As a result, rose and jasmine demand top dollar. On the other hand, peppermint is much less costly because the plant contains more essential oil, is relatively easy to grow and tend, and is harvested with machinery.

Many other factors, such as difficult growing conditions, the rarity of the plant, or where the plant is grown, affect essential oil prices. Surprisingly, cheaper oils will probably end up costing you more in the long run. Lesser quality oils are often weaker than high quality ones, and you will have to use more of them to achieve the same effect as a smaller amount of the high quality oil. Depending on how much more you have to use, you may end up spending more than if you'd simply purchased the better quality oil to begin with.

STORAGE

Once you've purchased quality essential oils, you certainly will want to keep them that way. Store them in glass containers. Some essential oils can actually dissolve plastic, and storing them even temporarily in it may contaminate the oil. Don't store essential oils in dropper bottles either, as it doesn't take long for the rubber seals and squeeze bulbs to melt into a gooey mess.

The color of the bottle doesn't really matter. Just be sure to keep all essential oils out of direct sunlight and away from heat so they don't lose their potency.

Essential oils are natural preservatives and will help preserve your carrier oils. Their scent will change and fade over time, however, and eventually lose its quality. Properly stored, most oils will keep for at least several years. The citrus oils, such as orange and lemon, are most vulnerable to losing their smell, but even they will keep for a couple of years if refrigerated.

A few essential oils, including patchouli, clary sage, benzoin, vetiver, and sandalwood, actually help fix the scent of other aromas combined with them. And they get better with age. The same is true for thick resins such as myrrh. Patchouli that has been stored for many years smells so rich, few people recognize it—even those who otherwise dislike it! Essential oils such as these become yet more valuable with age.

MAKE YOUR OWN MIXTURES

Making aromatherapy products to use for healing or as skin care products is as easy as it is fun. And you don't need much in the way of equipment to get started. In fact, you probably have most of what you need in your kitchen already. Add some bottles, some essential oils, and some carrier oils to your supplies and you'll be ready to begin experimenting.

SUPPLIES

A measuring cup, measuring spoons, and perhaps some small funnels will start you on the road to aromatherapy production. Unless you are adding essential oils to a ready-made product, you will need appropriate bottles or containers for storage. Simple bottles and vials are sold at drugstores; for fancier ones, check out your local natural food store. Mail order sources offer a greater variety of containers. Buy some labels for the bottles, too. Make sure to have paper towels and rubbing alcohol on hand for clean up.

You will need a way to measure small amounts of the essential oils and transfer them from bottle to bottle. Some essential oils are sold in bottles that have an insert called a reducer that allows only a drop of oil to come out at a time. It may take a few tries to get comfortable using it, but do not shake the bottle or several drops will come out at once. Glass droppers work well for obtaining just the right amount of essential oil and are sold in drugstores, some natural food stores, and by some essential oil suppliers.

MEASUREMENT CONVERSIONS

12.5 drops = 1/8 teaspoon = 1/48 oz = 1/6 dram = about 5/8 ml.

25 drops = 1/4 teaspoon = 1/24 oz = 1/3 dram = about 1 1/4 ml.

75 drops = 3/4 teaspoon = 1/8 oz = 1 dram = about 3.7 ml.

100 drops = 1 teaspoon = 1/6 oz = 1 1/3 dram = about 5 ml.

Be careful not to contaminate your essential oils by putting a dropper from one oil into another, but you don't need a separate dropper for each oil. Simply rinse the dropper in rubbing alcohol and wait a few minutes for the alcohol to completely evaporate before putting it into another oil. Having two or three droppers allows you to rotate them for rinsing and drying.

If you prefer, use a long, narrow tube called a pipette to measure out small amounts of essential oils. Pipettes can be made of glass or plastic; however, the easiest to use—but hardest to clean—is plastic with a squeeze bulb at one end. Practice with these using water before attempting to get exact measurements with your essential oils. Pipettes are sold in chemical equipment catalogs, some drugstores, and aromatherapy supply catalogs.

To measure larger quantities, use a Pyrex measuring cup with a pour spout. A set of measuring spoons is also useful for measuring more than a few drops of essential oil. In addition to the equipment, you'll also need some essential oils and various carriers such as vegetable oil, distilled water, rubbing alcohol, and vodka. You can buy or order fancier vegetable oils, such as almond, apricot, grape seed, and jojoba, at most natural food stores.

CARRIERS

Mixing your essential oil with a carrier oil is the most popular way of preparing aromatherapy products. It is also the easiest way to dilute essential oils in preparation for use. There are several choices of carriers; the most common are vegetable oil, alcohol, water, and more rarely, vinegar. The carrier you choose will depend on how you plan to apply your treatment. For a massage or body oil, vegetable oil is the best choice. For a liniment, you may prefer alcohol as your base because it doesn't leave an oily residue. A room spray only needs a water base, while aloe vera juice is perfect for a complexion spray.

You can also dilute essential oils in ready-made products that use vegetable oils as their base, such as salves, creams, or lotions that you purchase at the store. This is a quick way to custom-make your own products. Select products that have little or no essential oils in them already to ensure that you do not end up with too much scent in the finished product. Many natural food stores sell unscented cream, lotion, and shampoo bases.

BASIC ESSENTIAL OIL STARTER KIT

Lavender: fights infection, inflammation, insomnia, pain, depression, anxiety; appropriate for all complexion and hair types

Chamomile: aids digestion and promotes relaxation; treats allergies, menstrual cramps, depression, inflammation, anxiety, anger, rashes, and dry and problem skin, complexion, and hair

Rosemary: relieves pain, congestion, constipation and grief; stimulates circulation and memory; appropriate for most complexion and hair types

Tea Tree: fights most types of infection; appropriate for oily skin and hair

Peppermint: relieves indigestion, sinus congestion, itching, and panic; mental stimulant; use small amounts for dry skin and hair

Lemon, Orange, or other citrus: antidepressant; kills parasites; appropriate for oily complexion and hair

Geranium: balances mind and body; appropriate for all complexion and hair types

DILUTIONS

Most aromatherapy applications are a two-percent dilution. This means 2 drops of essential oil is added for every 100 drops of carrier oil, a safe and effective dilution for most aromatherapy applications. A one-percent dilution is suggested for children, pregnant women, and those who are weak from chronic illness. In some cases, you will want to use even less. Dilutions of three percent or more are used only for strong preparations such as liniments or for "spot" therapy, when you are only treating a tiny area instead of the entire body. Always remember that in aromatherapy, more is not necessarily better. In fact, too great a concentration may produce unwanted reactions. (Be sure to review the safety information in the next section.) The following are standard dilutions:

- **1 percent dilution: 5-6 drops per ounce of carrier**

- **2 percent dilution: 10-12 drops (about 1/8 teaspoon) per ounce of carrier**

- **3 percent dilution: 15-18 drops (a little less than 1/4 teaspoon) per ounce of carrier**

SAFETY

Essential oils are potent substances that can be harmful if mishandled. Unlike an herb tea or tincture that is made with the whole herb, essential oils are extremely concentrated.

Work with essential oils in a well-ventilated space, and take frequent breaks while handling them. Overexposure to an oil either through the skin or by smelling can result in nausea, headache, skin irritation, emotional unease, or a "spaced out" feeling. If you find yourself feeling like this, get some fresh air right away. If you experience skin irritation, quickly dilute the oil by applying straight vegetable oil to the affected area. Water won't be as effective since essential oils are not soluble in water.

Don't apply essential oils directly on the skin, referred to in aromatherapy as "neat," because of the danger of overdose. The gentler oils, such as lavender, may occasionally be used undiluted on a very small area, say an insect bite or skin eruption. But rubbing just a few drops of most essential oils directly onto the skin could easily amount to ingesting the equivalent of 10 cups of herb tea all at once! In addition to irritating or even burning your skin, you could damage your liver and kidneys, which must detoxify large amounts of essential oils once they enter the blood stream. Damage to the liver or kidneys is not always readily apparent, so you could be injuring your health without even knowing it.

Be especially careful when using essential oils known to be skin irritants (allspice, bay, cinnamon, clove, oregano, sage, savory, thyme [except linalol], thuja, and wintergreen). Never use these with children, the elderly, people who are very ill with a chronic disease, or anyone with liver or kidney damage, asthma, or a heart problem. Instead, turn to less harmful alternatives. A good example is thyme oil. Even diluted applications can burn the skin, so substitute lemon thyme, which is much milder. Oregano essential oil is so potent that many aromatherapists will not use it. Instead, they use the closely related marjoram or lavender, which are equal if not better muscle relaxants and antiseptics.

5 RECIPES TO TRY

Looking for a way to get started? Here are ten simple recipes you can try. You'll find more in the Common Conditions section at the back of the book.

FACIAL TONER FOR OILY COMPLEXIONS

12 drops lemongrass oil
6 drops juniper berry oil
2 drops ylang ylang oil
1 ounce witch hazel lotion
1 ounce aloe vera gel

Combine all of the ingredients in a glass bottle. Give the mixture a good shake and it's done! Apply at least once a day. If you find witch hazel too drying, vinegar is an excellent substitute. It is not as drying as the witch hazel lotion and helps to retain the skin's natural acid balance.

NASAL INHALER FOR SINUS CONGESTION

5 drops eucalyptus oil

¼ teaspoon coarse salt

Place the salt in a small vial (glass is best) with a tight lid and add essential oil. The salt will absorb the oil so it won't spill when you carry it. When needed, open the vial and inhale deeply. This same technique can be used with any essential oil listed above. Sniff as needed throughout the day.

DERMATITIS SKIN CARE

8 drops tea tree oil

8 drops chamomile oil

1 teaspoon Oregon grape tincture

2 ounces healing salve

With a toothpick, stir the tincture and essential oils into the salve. This will make the salve semi-liquid. You can purchase the tincture at a natural food store. Apply one to four times a day.

PICK-ME-UP COMBO

8 drops lemon oil

2 drops eucalyptus oil

2 drops peppermint oil

1 drop cinnamon leaf oil

1 drop cardamom oil (expensive, so optional)

2 ounces vegetable oil

Combine the ingredients. Use as a massage oil, add 2 teaspoons to your bath, or add 1 teaspoon to a footbath.

HEADACHE-BE-GONE COMPRESS

5 drops lavender or eucalyptus oil

1 cup cold water

Add essential oil to water, and swish a soft cloth in it. Wring out the cloth, lie down, and close your eyes. Place the cloth over your forehead and eyes. Use throughout the day, as often as you can.

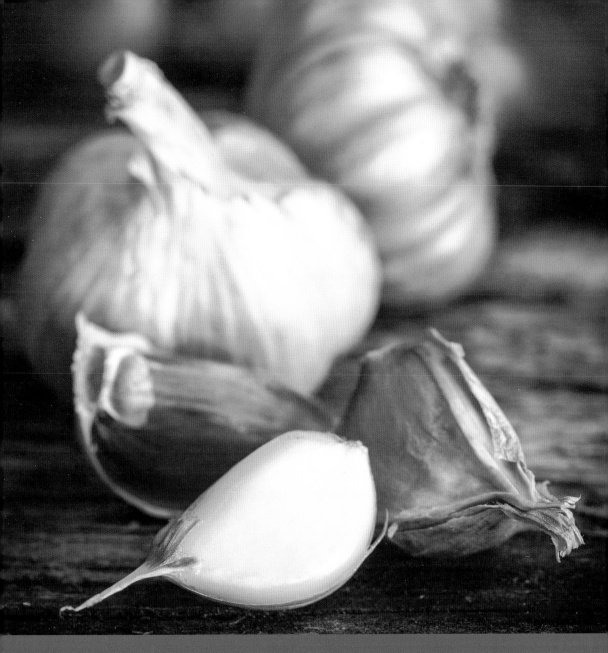

KITCHEN CURE-ALLS

Today, we think of garlic, vinegar, olive oil, and honey as staples of our kitchen and pantry. But throughout history, these foods haven't just been used to add flavor, but to increase health. Let's take a new look at these traditional cures.

GARLIC

Garlic, or scientifically speaking, *Allium sativum*, is cultivated across the globe except in the polar regions. The bulb of this attractive plant contains more powerful sulfur compounds than does any other *Allium* species, such as onions and leeks. The garlic plant may have evolved to include these smelly sulfur compounds as a way of warding off foraging animals, invasive insects, and even soil-borne microorganisms such as bacteria and fungi. Yet these same compounds, which lend garlic its pungent aroma and delectable flavor as well as its medicinal qualities, are exactly the reason so many people are attracted to the bulb.

FABLES AND FOLKLORE

Garlic, which has been grown for more than 5,000 years, is one of the oldest cultivated plants in the world. Researchers think the ancient Egyptians were the first to farm garlic; in fact, the little bulbs helped power the building of the great pyramids.

Ancient Egyptians bestowed many sacred qualities upon garlic. They believed it kept away evil spirits, so they buried garlic-shape lumps of clay with dead pharaohs. Archaeologists found preserved bulbs of garlic scattered around King Tut's tomb millennia after his burial. The ancient Egyptians believed so strongly in the power of garlic to ward off evil spirits that they would chew it before making a journey at night. Garlic made them burp and gave them foul-smelling breath, creating a radius of odor so strong, they believed, that evil spirits would not penetrate it.

Ancient Greeks and Romans loved their garlic, too. Greek athletes and soldiers ate garlic before entering the arena or battlefield because they thought it had strength-enhancing properties. Roman soldiers ate garlic for inspiration and courage. Greek midwives hung garlic cloves in birthing rooms to repel evil spirits. Hippocrates, the ancient Greek known as the "father of medicine," prescribed garlic for a variety of ailments around 400 B.C. It was used to treat wounds, fight infection, cure leprosy, and ease digestive disorders. Other prominent Greeks used garlic to treat heart problems, as well.

Garlic's reputation as a medicinal wonder continued into the Middle Ages. It was used in attempts to prevent the plague and to treat leprosy and a long list of other ailments. Later, explorers and migrating peoples introduced this easy-to-grow and easy-to-carry plant to various regions around the world. The Spanish, Portuguese, and French introduced garlic to the Americas.

In many historic cultures, garlic was used medicinally but not in cooking. That might surprise us today, but were our ancestors able to travel into the future to visit us, they would likely think us rather dense for our culture's general lack of appreciation for the bulb's healing qualities. Traditionally, garlic bulbs were prepared in a variety of ways for medicinal purposes. The juice of the bulb might be extracted and taken internally for one purpose, while the bulb might be ground into a paste for external treatment of other health problems.

IN RECENT HISTORY

Garlic played its first starring role in modern medical treatment during World War I. The Russians used garlic on the front lines to treat battle wounds and fight infection, and medics used moss that was soaked in garlic as an antiseptic to pack wounds.

In the first part of the 20th century, garlic saw plenty of action off the battlefield, too. Even though penicillin was discovered in 1928, the demand for it among the general population often outstripped the supply, so many people reverted to treatments they had used with some success before, including garlic.

The pungent, ancient remedy has found its way to modern times. Herbalists have long touted garlic for a number of health problems, from preventing colds and treating intestinal problems to lowering blood cholesterol and reducing heart-disease risk. Garlic remedies abound—and scientific research has begun to support the usefulness of some of them. Garlic's popularity today is due in part to the efforts of scientists around the world. They have identified a number of sulfur-containing compounds in garlic that have important medicinal properties.

INFECTION FIGHTER

One of garlic's most important roles is that of infection fighter. Laboratory studies confirm that raw garlic has antibacterial and antiviral properties. Not only does it knock out many common cold and flu viruses but its effectiveness also spans a broad range of both gram-positive and gram-negative bacteria (two major classifications of bacteria), fungus, intestinal parasites, and yeast. Cooking garlic, however, destroys the allicin, so you'll need to use raw garlic to prevent or fight infections.

One folk remedy is to battle colds and chest congestion with a garlic poultice or plaster. To make one, put some chopped garlic in a clean cloth, thin washcloth, or paper towel. Fold it over to enclose the garlic. Pour very warm (but not hot) water over the wrapped garlic, let it sit for a few seconds, and then lightly wring it out. Place the wrapped garlic on the chest for several minutes. Reheat with very warm water and place on the back, over the lung area, for several minutes. Some herbalists also recommend placing the poultice on the soles of the feet. Caution: Be careful not to let garlic come into direct contact with the skin. Cut garlic is so powerful that prolonged exposure to the skin may result in a burn.

Applying a topical solution of raw garlic and water may stop wounds from getting infected. (Simply crush one clove of garlic and mix it with one-third of a cup of clean water. Use the solution within three hours because it will lose its potency over time.) A garlic solution used as a footbath several times a day is traditionally believed to improve athlete's foot.

FOUR THIEVES' VINEGAR

There are about as many versions of the four thieves' vinegar story as there are recipes for the concoction. One popular version, reported to be from the Parliament of Toulouse archives of 1628–1631, goes like this: Four thieves living in Marseilles, France, during the 17th century plagues were convicted of going to the houses of plague victims and robbing them, but the thieves themselves never became ill. How was this possible? In order to get a lesser sentence they revealed their secret—they protected themselves by consuming daily doses of a mixture that contained vinegar, garlic, and a handful of other herbs. Those in charge were so grateful that they hanged the four thieves, rather than burning them at the stake. That's gratitude for you!

GARLIC'S ANTI-INFLAMMATORY PROPERTIES

Inflammation is the body's reaction to an injury, irritation, or infection. The symptoms of inflammation include redness, swelling, and pain. Whenever the body suffers an injury, it sends many substances to the site to begin the healing process and to fight off foreign invaders, such as bacteria that can cause infections. Inflammation is so vigorous in its duties that sometimes the surrounding tissues get damaged. This can occur at the site of a wound, inside blood vessels that have succumbed to an injury by oxidized LDL cholesterol, or in airways that are exposed to something that irritates them.

Certain complexes in garlic appear to help minimize the body's inflammatory response. By decreasing inflammation, garlic may lend a hand by doing the following:

- Protecting the inside of your arteries

- Reducing the severity of asthma

- Protecting against inflammation in the joints, such as in rheumatoid arthritis and osteoarthritis

- Reducing inflammation in nasal passages and airways, such as that associated with colds.

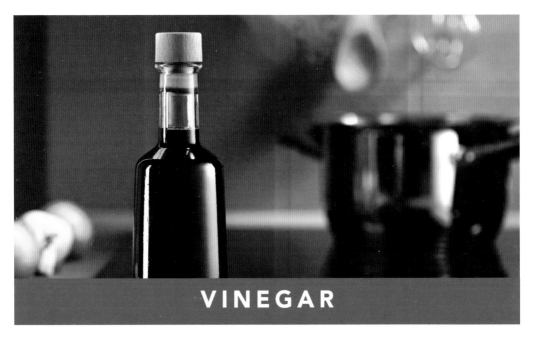

VINEGAR

Vinegar has been valued for its healing properties for about as long as garlic has, and like garlic, vinegar has found its way from the apothecary's shelf to the cook's pot. Today, it can continue to play that dual role, taking the place of less healthful dietary ingredients and helping to regulate blood sugar levels while entertaining our taste buds with its tart flavor.

FROM ANCIENT TIMES

The first vinegar was the result of an ancient accident. Once upon a time, a keg of wine (presumably a poorly sealed one that allowed oxygen in) was stored too long, and when the would-be drinkers opened it, they found a sour liquid instead of wine. The name "vinegar" is derived from the French words for "sour wine."

Fortunately, our resourceful ancestors found ways to use the "bad" wine. They put it to work as a cure-all, a food preservative, and later, a flavor enhancer. It wasn't long before they figured out how to make vinegar on purpose, and producing it became one of the world's earliest commercial industries.

The use of vinegar as medicine probably started soon after it was discovered. Its healing virtues are extolled in records of the Babylonians, and the great Greek physician Hippocrates reportedly used it as an antibiotic. Ancient Greek doctors poured vinegar into wounds and over dressings as a disinfectant, and they gave concoctions of honey and vinegar to patients recovering from illness. In Asia, early samurai warriors believed vinegar to be a tonic that would increase their strength and vitality.

VINEGAR TODAY

Vinegar continued to be used as a medicine in more recent times. During the Civil War and World War I, for example, military medics used vinegar to treat wounds. And folk traditions around the world still espoused vinegar for a wide variety of ailments. Natural-healing enthusiasts and vinegar fans continue to honor and use many of those folk remedies.

The folk- and natural-healing claims made for vinegar through the ages have been almost as plentiful and varied as those made for garlic. Even in the current era of high-tech medicine, some proponents of natural healing still encourage traditional uses of vinegar. Present-day vinegar fans view it as an overall health-boosting, disease-fighting tonic and recommend mixing a teaspoon or tablespoon of cider vinegar with a glass of water and drinking it each morning or before meals. (Apple cider vinegar is the traditional vinegar of choice for home or folk remedies, although some recent claims have been made for the benefits of wine vinegars, especially red wine vinegar.)

TRADITIONAL REMEDIES

You may want to give these traditional vinegar remedies a try:

Stomach upset. To settle minor stomach upset, try a simple cider vinegar tonic with a meal. Drinking a mixture of a spoonful of vinegar in a glass of water is said to improve digestion and ease minor stomach upset by stimulating digestive juices.

Common cold symptoms. Apple cider vinegar is also an age-old treatment for symptoms of the common cold. For a sore throat, mix one teaspoon of apple cider vinegar into a glass of water; gargle with a mouthful of the solution and then swallow it, repeating until you've finished all the solution in the glass. For a natural cough syrup, mix half a tablespoon apple cider vinegar with half a tablespoon honey and swallow. Finally, you can add a quarter-cup of apple cider vinegar to the recommended amount of water in your room vaporizer to help with congestion.

Itching or stinging from minor insect bites. In the folklore of New England, rural Indiana, and parts of the Southwest, a vinegar wash is sometimes used for treating bites and stings. (However, if the person bitten has a known allergy to insect venom or begins to exhibit signs of a serious allergic reaction, such as widespread hives, swelling of the face or mouth, difficulty breathing, or loss of consciousness, skip the home remedies and seek immediate medical attention.) Pour undiluted vinegar over the bite or sting, avoiding surrounding healthy skin as much as possible.

Athlete's foot. One way to eliminate athlete's foot (or other fungal infection) is to create an environment that is inhospitable to the fungus that causes the condition. The Amish traditionally use a footbath of vinegar and water to discourage the growth of athlete's foot fungus. To try this remedy, mix one cup of vinegar into two quarts of water in a basin or pan. Soak your feet in this solution every night for 15 to 30 minutes, using a fresh solution each night. Or, if you prefer, mix up a solution using one cup of vinegar and one cup of water. Apply the solution to the affected parts of your feet with a cotton ball. Let your feet dry completely before putting on socks and/or shoes.

VINEGAR AND DIABETES?

Vinegar has recently won attention for its potential to help people with type 2 diabetes get a better handle on their condition. A study cited in 2004 in the American Diabetes Association's publication *Diabetes Care* indicates that vinegar holds real promise for helping people with diabetes. In the study, 21 people with either type 2 diabetes or insulin resistance (a prediabetes condition) and eight control subjects were each given a solution containing five teaspoons of vinegar, five teaspoons of water, and one teaspoon of saccharin two minutes before ingesting a high-carbohydrate meal. The blood sugar and insulin levels of the participants were measured before the meal and 30 minutes and 60 minutes after the meal.

Vinegar increased overall insulin sensitivity 34 percent in the study participants who were insulin-resistant and 19 percent in those with type 2 diabetes. That means their bodies actually became more receptive to insulin, allowing the hormone to do its job of getting sugar out of the blood and into the cells. Both blood sugar and blood insulin levels were lower than normal in the insulin-resistant participants, which is more good news.

More studies certainly need to be done to confirm the extent of vinegar's benefits for type 2 diabetes patients and those at risk of developing this increasingly common disease. But for now, people with type 2 diabetes might be wise to talk with their doctors or dietitians about consuming more vinegar.

VINEGAR FOR FLAVOR

There are some delicious varieties of vinegar available. Each bestows a different taste or character to foods. The diversity and intensity of flavor are key to one important healing role that vinegar can play. Whether you are trying to protect yourself from cardiovascular diseases, such as heart disease, high blood pressure, or stroke, or you have been diagnosed with one or more of these conditions and have been advised to clean up your diet, vinegar should become a regular cooking and dining companion. That's because a tasty vinegar can often be used in place of sodium and/or ingredients high in saturated or trans fats to add flavor and excitement to a variety of dishes. Use vinegar for flavor as a substitute for mayonnaise in coleslaw, cream-based salad dressings on salads, or ketchup on fries.

OLIVE OIL

A diet that is rich in olive oil has enhanced the health of people living in the Mediterranean region for thousands of years. Within the past century, however, olive oil's benefits have also been scientifically investigated and acknowledged. This liquid gold works to keep hearts healthy, may reduce inflammation and the risk of certain cancers, and might even play a role in controlling diabetes and weight.

IN ANTIQUITY

Many theories exist as to where olive trees originated, but one that is fairly well accepted is that they first grew in Asia Minor, the land bridge between Europe and

Asia that is now home to Turkey and Syria. Evidence shows that humans in this area were using olives more than 8,000 years ago. Historians believe olive use spread throughout the rest of the Mediterranean region about 6,000 years ago. Phoenicians carried olive trees to what is now southern Europe, as well as to Egypt and other areas along the North African coast. Like garlic, olive remnants have been found inside Egyptian tombs, signifying the important role they played in that culture.

Later, the Greeks and Romans put olives to good use. People in both of these ancient civilizations used olive oil to counteract poisons and to treat open wounds, insect bites, headaches, and stomach and digestive problems. They also applied olive oil to the body before bathing (it functioned as soap) and then again afterward to moisturize the skin and to form a barrier against dirt and the sun's rays. The Romans took olives along in their travels, planting them wherever they went and spreading their beneficial qualities to many regions.

FOLK REMEDIES

As the olive migrated, folk remedies that used olive oil evolved to reflect the times and maladies of different regions. Olive oil was taken by mouth, spread on the skin, and dropped into the ears or nose. People considered it both a cure and a preventative measure for many afflictions. Here are some popular folk remedies that have been used over the years:

- Take a spoonful or two to treat an upset stomach, difficult digestion, or constipation or to reduce the body's absorption of alcohol from alcoholic beverages.

- Apply to skin to prevent dryness and wrinkles, to soften the skin, and to treat acne.

- Use on the hair to make it shiny and to treat dandruff.

- Strengthen nails by soaking them in warm olive oil.

- Ease aching muscles by massaging them with olive oil.

- Lower blood pressure by boiling olive tree leaves and drinking the "tea."

- Clear nasal congestion with drops of olive oil in the nose.

A word of caution: Using olive oil as a folk remedy may not be safe for children. You should always consult a pediatrician before trying any treatment—whether folk remedy or over-the-counter drug—on a child.

A HEALTHY LIFESTYLE

Chronic diseases and conditions that are caused, in part, by unhealthy foods and sedentary lifestyles plague many societies today, especially those in the Western world. The good news is that olive oil, which contains healthy fat, may help with the worst of them, including heart disease, hypertension (high blood pressure), metabolic syndrome, inflammation, cancer, diabetes, and problems associated with obesity.

So whether or not you use olive oil as a folk remedy, try to incorporate it in your diet for good results!

HONEY

If you're used to using honey as a flavoring for tea and not much else, you won't bee-lieve the many medicinal benefits of honey! From soothing burns and bug bites to treating upset tummies, honey has you covered.

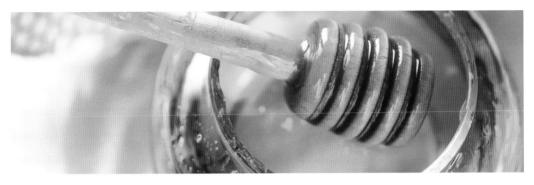

HONEY HISTORY

Ancient Egyptians used honey as a form of payment, similar to the way Aztecs used cocoa beans. They also used honey to feed the animals they considered sacred, and offered honey as a tribute to the gods. Several giant vats of honey, untouched for more than 3,000 years, were excavated from King Tut's tomb. Incredibly, the honey was found to still be edible.

Hippocrates, known as the father of modern medicine, was the first to write about the medicinal properties of honey (circa 460–377 B.C.). He discovered that honey is beneficial to one's complexion. He believed that honey is an expectorant, adds heat to the body, and is beneficial for healing ulcers.

Not too long ago, in the pre-penicillin era, doctors serving in World War II treated burns and wounds with honey. Today, honey can still be used as a folk remedy.

SAFETY NOTE

Although honey is naturally free of allergens, never feed honey to children younger than 1 year of age. Their underdeveloped digestive systems cannot attack certain bacterial spores. This can result in infant botulism, a rare but serious disease that affects infants' nervous systems.

HOW HONEY CAN HELP

Coat a minor burn with honey to soothe the pain, reduce inflammation, get rid of bacteria, and reduce burn marks.

Take the sting out of bug bites. Combine honey with enough ground cinnamon to form a paste, and apply it to the site of an insect bite to reduce the pain, irritation, and itchiness.

You may be able to **fend off a migraine** if you feel one coming on. Just take 1 teaspoon of honey as soon as you feel the warning signs. If it's already too late, take 2 teaspoons of honey with each meal until the headache subsides.

Sore throats respond well to this drink: In a glass of water, mix 1 teaspoon honey, 3 tablespoons lime juice, and 1 tablespoon pineapple juice. Sip to obtain soothing relief.

Bye-bye, bad breath. Stir equal parts honey and vinegar into a glass of water, gargle, and rinse. For good measure, use a toothbrush to remove any remaining residue.

Digest this suggestion: A teaspoon or two of honey mixed with milk can help improve digestion. The mixture works well either warm or cold, but some people swear by warm milk.

Obtain relief from a hangover by taking 1 teaspoon honey every hour until you feel better. The large quantity of fructose found in honey will help speed up the metabolism of alcohol in your system.

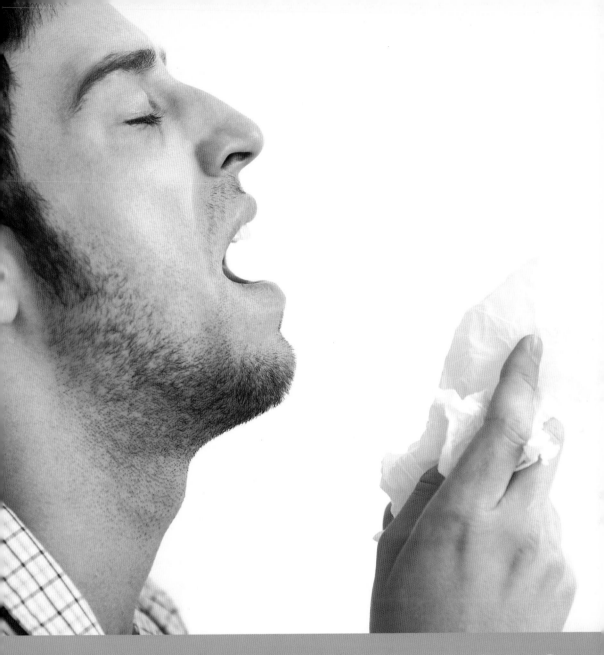

COMMON CONDITIONS

In this section we'll explore some traditional methods from around the world for helping, easing, or curing some common conditions that many people experience throughout their lifetime.

BITES AND STINGS

When bees, wasps, and other insects bite or sting you, they may release a poison-ous venom that produces pain, swelling, redness, itching, or burning. Most people recover from a bee or wasp sting in a couple of hours. About three percent of the population develops an allergic reaction called anaphylaxis, in which painful hives erupt and swelling blocks airways, leading to circulatory collapse and even death. If you've had an allergic response in the past, discuss the matter with your doctor, and make plans for how to deal with another bite or sting in the future.

Here are some traditional aids to ease the pain.

Smother it with onion. A homegrown Amish remedy for bee stings is to apply a freshly cut onion *(Allium cepa)*. Hold the onion slice on the wound for at least ten minutes, then discard.

Smear on some baking supplies. Who'd have thought that a couple of kitchen staples could take the bite out of a bee sting? Well, someone, at some time, came up with this traditional folk remedy. Mix one tablespoon each of vinegar and baking soda. Apply the paste, and leave it on the sting as long as possible. Apply more, if necessary.

Try some tobacco. But don't smoke or chew it if you want to stay healthy! Instead, apply it to bug bites and stings in a traditional poultice. Maya Indians used wild tobacco *(Nicotiana rustica, N. glauca)*, moistened with saliva, to treat bee stings. In a case of parallel development, this unlikely remedy was also employed by the Six Nations, a league of Indians extending from the Hudson River to Lake Erie. In some parts of Appalachia today, tobacco poultices are still used to heal bee, hornet, yellow jacket, wasp, and spider bites and stings.

Ice an itch. Itchy mosquito bites may benefit from an ice-cold compress. Ice the bite for 20 minutes at a time every few hours. The same goes for nonpoisonous spider bites, which can also leave an itchy welt.

Go for the garlic. Garlic contains broad-spectrum antibiotic and anti-inflammatory substances that can disinfect and soothe a bite or sting. Crush a clove of garlic and mix it with a little water to form a paste, and then apply the paste directly to the sting area.

COLDS AND FLU

The common cold is aptly named. It is so common, in fact, that all human beings from every region of the globe experience it at one time or another during their lives. A simple common cold is a collection of familiar symptoms signalling an infection of the upper respiratory tract, which includes the nose, throat, and sinuses. Many different types of viruses cause colds.

Although we often say "colds and flu" in the same breath, influenza is a very different disease from the common cold. The influenza virus takes up residence mainly in the throat and bronchial tract. The flu usually comes accompanied by a fever, which is not usually present in a cold. The fever generally passes within a few days, but the fatigue, muscle aches, and cough that result from the flu can linger for weeks.

In general, remedies for the cold and flu focus on boosting the immune system and managing the symptoms.

Follow the plains. For centuries, Plains Indians used purple coneflower, or Echinacea *(Echinacea angustifolia, Echinacea purpurea)*, as a remedy for colds and flu. It's become one of the best-selling herbal remedies in the country. While studies suggest that Echinacea activates the immune system, scientists don't completely understand how. You can purchase a tincture of Echinacea at a health-food store or drugstore. Take it off at the first sign of a cold or flu to stave off the worst of the effects.

Eat like an ancient Egyptian. The recommendation to take garlic *(Allium sativan)* for colds comes from New England, the American Southwest, and all the way from China. Garlic has been used for colds, bronchial problems, and fevers in cultures throughout the world since the dawn of written medical history. Even the ancient Egyptians used it to treat cough and fever.

Blend three cloves of garlic in a blender with a little water. (The clove must be cut or crushed to release its constituents.) If you want, add half a lemon, skin and all, to the garlic. Put the contents in a cup and fill the cup with boiling water. Let steep for five minutes, inhaling the fragrance. Strain, add honey, and drink the entire cup in sips. Do this two to three times a day while you have a cold or flu, or once a day to prevent infection during epidemics.

Take advantage of a rural remedy. Onions, cousins to garlic, have also been used to treat colds in virtually every folk tradition in North America, whether eaten raw, roasted, or boiled; taken in the form of teas, milk, or even wine; worn in a sock or in a bag around the neck; or applied to the chest as a poultice. Wild onions have been used for the same purpose by Native American tribes throughout the country. Using onions to treat colds persists today in the folk medicine or New England, North Carolina, Indiana, and Appalachia. Perhaps because the onion's pungent aroma seems to cut through even the stuffiest nose, cold sufferers have been drawn to the bulb and its anti-infective properties.

To see for yourself, cut up one large onion and simmer in a covered pot for twenty minutes. Drink a cup of the tea three or four times daily when you have a cold or flu.

ONION SYRUP FOR A COUGH

Slice a raw onion, put it in a bowl, and then cover the onion slices with sugar. Allow the onion to sit at room temperature until syrup forms. You don't need to add water because the sugar sucks the juice out of the onion. It may take a day or two for the syrup to form naturally; you can speed up the process by putting the sugar-covered onions in the oven and baking them at a medium heat until the syrup forms. Take a tablespoon of the onion syrup several times a day. The syrup will last for a day or two; make a new, fresh batch if the cough lasts longer than that.

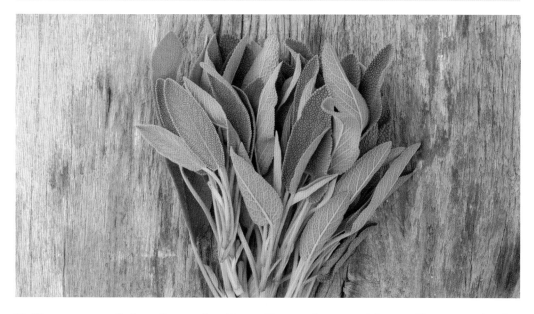

Follow sage advice from the East Coast. Some residents of New England, North Carolina, and Indiana recommend hot sage *(Salvia officinalis)* tea to "break up" a cold. They say sage is especially good for sore throats. Place one teaspoon of sage in a cup and fill with boiling water. Cover and let steep for ten minutes. Strain, add a little lemon and honey, and drink. Repeat three to four times a day as long as the cold lasts.

Do as the Romans. The contemporary folk traditions of New England and Indiana call for drinking hot lemonade during a cold or flu, but the practice is at least as old as the ancient Romans. To make this time-tested potion, place one chopped, whole lemon—skin, pulp, and all—in a pot, and add one cup of boiling water. While letting the mixture steep for five minutes, inhale the fumes. Then strain and drink. Do this at the onset of a cold, and repeat three to four times a day for the duration of a cold.

Follow the wisdom of Hippocrates. Inhaling the fumes of vinegar is a cold remedy as old as ancient Greece. The famous physician Hippocrates recommended the treatment for coughs and respiratory infections. In a jar, pour half a cup of boiling water over half a cup of vinegar. Gently inhale the steam, being careful not to burn yourself.

Turn to salt. The remedy of sniffing salt water to ease nasal congestion is part of New England and Indiana folk medicine and is even often recommended by conventional medical doctors. Ayurvedic physicians from India use a special pot, called a neti, to make the process easier. To help yourself breathe easier, put a quarter teaspoon of salt in a glass of hot or warm water, and sniff some of the water. (Make sure you're using distilled, sterile water.) Do this after being exposed to someone with a cold or flu, or at the first sign of infection. Repeat every three to four hours while suffering from a cold.

You can also try gargling with warm salt water (a quarter teaspoon salt in four ounces warm water) every one to two hours to soothe your sore throat.

Try buttering yourself up. Adding butter to hot tea is a remedy used in the high altitudes of Nepal and Tibet to prevent colds. Add one tablespoon of butter to a cup of hot tea. Let the butter melt, so that it forms a thin layer across the top of the tea.

Drink a glass of tea. Folk traditions often advise a cold or flu sufferer to sip hot, fragrant teas. Most herbs used to treat colds (including elder, ginger, yarrow, mint, thyme, lemon balm, catnip, garlic, onion, and mustard) contain aromatic oils that are believed to produce antibacterial, antivirual, antifungal, and anti-inflammatory actions. The oils escape with the steam of the hot tea.

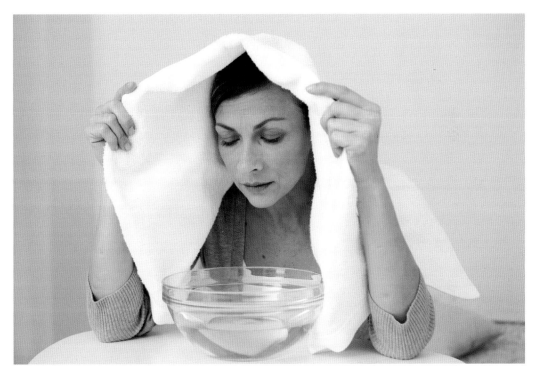

Get steamed. Speaking of steam, you can inhale steam from essential oils of sage, hyssop, thyme, lavender, or eucalyptus. Add a few drops of one or more oils to a bowl of hot water. Lean over the bowl with a towel draped over your head and inhale deeply.

Heat it up. To relieve sinus pain and congestion, try drinking a cup of tea made with lemon and ginger or horseradish to which you've added a dash or two of cayenne pepper.

Try a tonic. This home remedy dates back about 150 years, and soothes both body and soul. Do not give it to children younger than two, however, as honey can cause infant botulism and allergic reactions in children.

Mix one tablespoon of honey and one tablespoon of apple cider vinegar with eight ounces of hot water. Use as often as desired. You can also substitute lemon juice for apple cider vinegar.

Pull out the flannel. To soothe a sore throat, mix two cups of hot water with two drops of lavender oil, two drops of bergamot oil, and one drop of tea tree oil. Soak a cloth—flannel works best—in the liquid, wring it out, and wrap the cloth around your throat.

Suck on a lemon. Another sore throat remedy is to suck a lemon sprinkled with salt. Another variation is to mix lemon juice with water-diluted salt.

Listen to the singers. For centuries, singers from European countries have gargled with marjoram tea sweetened with honey.

Rub it in. This homemade vapor rub helps ease congestion. Gather 12 drops eucalyptus oil, 5 drops peppermint oil, 5 drops thyme oil, and 1 ounce olive oil. Combine ingredients in a glass bottle. Shake well to mix oils evenly. Gently massage into chest and throat. Use one to five times per day, especially just before bed.

Quiet a cough. To help break up chest congestion and soothe a cough, try a nightcap of anise-seed tea. Crush 2 teaspoons anise seeds, steep in a cup of boiling water for ten minutes, strain, and drink the tea just before hitting the hay.

WHAT ABOUT CHICKEN SOUP?

One of the most beneficial hot fluids you can consume when you have a cold is chicken soup. It's been used as a remedy for the common cold for a long time—back to rabbi/physician Moses Maimonides in twelfth-century Egypt! In 1978, Marvin Sackner, M.D., of Mount Sinai Hospital in Miami Beach, Florida, included chicken soup in a test of the effects of sipping hot and cold water on the clearance of mucus. Chicken soup placed first, hot water second, and cold water a distant third. Sackner's work has since been replicated by other researchers. While doctors aren't sure exactly why chicken soup helps clear nasal passages, they agree it helps.

CUTS AND BRUISES

Everyone gets their share of small cuts and bruises. Cleanliness is important, since even the smallest scratch can become infected. Here are some time-tested ways to treat small wounds. Note that if you have diabetes or circulation issues, you should consult your doctor on the best ways to treat wounds.

Packs, potatoes, and peels. There are several handy treatments that can be applied to a cut that's about to turn into a bruise. One is to wrap a cold pack in a thin dish towel and place it on the affected area as soon after the injury occurs as possible. Leave it on for a good twenty minutes. Another treatment, favored by farmers throughout the years, is to place a thin slice of raw potato on the bump as soon as possible and leave it there until the pain subsides. The third option simply involves substituting a banana peel for the raw potato; apply the inside of the peel to the skin. All three of these fixes have anti-inflammatory properties that will speed healing, and the banana skin is also said to reduce discoloration.

Make a mash. If you don't act quickly enough and a bruise does develop, try speeding it away by covering the area with a mash of crushed fresh parsley leaves. Apply the crushed parsley a few times in the day or two after the bruise appears to speed healing.

Sage for canker sores. Canker sores are small round or oval ulcers that occur inside the mouth, on the tongue, or on the lower part of the gums. They are painful but typically harmless and noncontagious. (They are not to be confused with cold sores, which are painful and contagious lesions that occur on the outer surface of the lips.) To get relief from a canker sore, steep 2 teaspoons ground sage seasoning in hot water for ten minutes. All to cool a bit, then add ½ teaspoon lemon juice and gargle with the solution.

Tea tree oil for infection. Clean any cut or scratch with soap and water to ward off infection. Then apply tea tree oil to help prevent infection. Reapply twice a day for up to 7 days. Tea tree oil is a natural antiseptic.

Go for sweet relief. Raw honey can be applied to a minor cut or scrape to serve as an emergency anti-infective ointment. It's been used to help protest wounds since ancient times.

EYE PROBLEMS

Inflammations of the eye can be painful and produce redness, swelling, and irritation. Conjunctivitis, or pinkeye, is an inflammation of the conjunctiva, the delicate

membrane that lines the inner curve of the eyelid and covers the exposed surface of
the eye. The infection results from disease-causing microorganisms, such as bacteria,
fungi, and viruses. Eye inflammation also may be caused by allergies, chemicals, dust,
smoke, and foreign objects that become lodged in the eye. Conventional treatment
varies according to cause and symptoms. Doctors may prescribe antibiotics, steroids,
or soothing eyedrops. And of course most of us have experienced simple eyestrain
from looking at an electronic screen for too long. Here are some fixes for tired,
strained, or reddened eyes.

How about a spot of tea? Tea is a common eye remedy, from Appalachia to India and other Asian countries. It's easy if you use black- or green-tea bags. Prepare tea
according to the directions. Then place the tea bag on your closed eye for 15 minutes. Repeat as needed. Meanwhile, sip away.

A sweet smelling remedy. A rose is a rose is a…cure for infected eyes, as they
might say in Spanish- and Arabic-speaking communities. If you have access to roses
that are free of pesticides and other chemicals, place a handful of petals in a jar and
add one pint of boiling water. Cover well to retain the aromatic oils and let stand
until the water has cooled to room temperature. Strain, then soak a clean cloth with
the liquid and place on the closed eye.

Apply an Incan poultice. This unlikely cure comes from the Inca. The Inca cultivated potatoes for food and medicine, and one medical use included eye conditions.
Remove the skin from a whole raw potato and grate finely. Place the grated potato
in a clean cloth and fold to make a poultice. Apply to your eye for 15 minutes.

Give yourself flowers. In Asia, chrysanthemum blossoms make a great remedy
for tired, aching eyes. Place a large handful of flowers in a pot and add one quart of
boiling water. Cover and steep for ten minutes, and then strain. The wet flowers are

wrapped in a clean cloth. Then, the poultice is placed on the eye while the patient sips the tea.

Calm them with chamomile. Aromatherapists recommend a chamomile cure for tired eyes. Steep two chamomile tea bags in a few tablespoons of hot water. Allow the bags to cool somewhat. Then lie down and place a tea bag over each eye. Cover the poultices with a soft cloth.

Try a Tibetan tip. In Tibet, a tea made of fennel is used to soothe tired, irritated eyes.

Buy a plant. If you have dry eyes, increasing the humidity in your home or office can help. Using a humidifier is an obvious way to do this. But setting a pot of water on your home radiator can also increase the humidity level in your home. Potted plants in your home or office can also act as inexpensive—and attractive—humidifiers.

FATIGUE, STRESS, AND ANXIETY

When our lives our busy and stressful, we often experience physical responses, from fatigue to insomnia to muscle tension. If you're tired, irritable, or stressed out, here are some tips that may help.

Repeat yourself. Select a word or sound that is pleasing to you, and say it over and over again to yourself with your eyes closed. In India, devotees of meditation call this a mantra. Chanting your word or phrase long enough has calming effects.

Follow the Pied Piper's lead. Legend has it that the Pied Piper of storybook fame lured the rats away from Hamelin by enticing them with valerian, an herb whose pungent odor reminds many people of dirty socks. Nonetheless, valerian tea is one of the plant world's most powerful sedatives. Folk healers in Europe have prescribed the herb for sleeplessness for centuries. However, be aware that for some people, valerian actually causes agitation, so if you experience that side effect, do not persist.

Sniff a sprig of lavender. Aromatherapists say the essential oil produced by this lovely garden plant works wonders to ease jangled nerves.

Squeeze your thumb. Practitioners of jin shin jyutsu, a Japanese touch-based therapy based on the principles of acupuncture, link various emotions with each finger. Worry is said to be the domain of the thumb. Press it gently until you feel yourself relaxing.

Swallow a bitter pill. Bitters are the 19th-century remedy that some German physicians still prescribe today. Bitter tonics are made from plants with a strong bitter flavor, but the medicines are not strong themselves. In fact, many act as mild sedatives and act to cure fatigue. The most famous bitter herbs in North America are goldthread, goldenseal, Oregon grape root, yellow dock, dandelion root, and betony.

ROSEMARY TEA RECIPE

It is said that rosemary can raise energy levels. Add a few sprigs to your bath or sip a cup of rosemary tea.

To make tea, steep one teaspoon of rosemary in one cup hot water for fifteen minutes. Drink up to three cups a day.

Get prodded out of your fatigue. According to practitioners of Chinese medicine, an insufficiency of qi, the body's vital force, can cause myriad symptoms, including fatigue. Acupuncture and moxibustion are used to bring energy to deficient organs and systems. Acupuncture is also used to treat insomnia, another side-effect of stress and anxiety.

Borrow your kitty's catnip. If you're suffering some insomnia, reach for catnip tea. Catnip, a common weed that makes felines go bonkers, helps some people to fall asleep.

Sleep with an Old World cure. Stuffing a pillow with soothing herbs with soothing herbs is an old European remedy for sleeplessness. Many people in the United States use herb pillows today—you can buy them or make your own. Children should sleep on pillows filled with mild herbs, such as lavender, lemon balm, chamomile, and dill. Adults may prefer pillows stuffed with hop, the herb that gives beer its bitter flavor.

UPLIFTING FORMULA

6 drops bergamot oil
3 drops petitgrain oil
3 drops geranium oil
1 drop neroli (expensive, so optional)
2 ounces vegetable oil

Combine all the ingredients. Use as a massage oil, add 1 or 2 teaspoons to your bath, or add 1 teaspoon to a foot bath. For an equally uplifting room or facial spritzer, substitute the same amount of water for the vegetable oil in this formula. Put the water formula in a spray bottle, or spritz and sniff throughout the day as needed.

FEVER

The body's normal temperature is around 98.6 degrees Fahrenheit, although that temperature can fluctuate depending on the person and the time of day. To qualify as a fever, the temperature usually has to top 100 degrees. A fever is a symptom of infection, such as flu, measles, or another ailment, ranging from dehydration to heart attack. Symptoms may accompany fever, including headache, thirst, redness of the face, chills, and mental confusion.

Ease it with oil. Some essential oils will cool you off. Apply or inhale bergamot, chamomile, or eucalyptus.

Get cold feet. Reactive hydrotherapy is a practice taught in North American naturopathic colleges. Soak cotton socks in cold water, wring them out, and place them on the patient's feet. Cover the cold socks with one or two pairs of warm wool socks and leave in place for about 40 minutes.

Take a tip from Tibet. Tibetan physicians prescribe several herbs for reducing fever, including white sandalwood, fennel, and scute.

Sweat it out. Sweating cools the body during a fever, and many traditional folk remedies use herbs to encourage it. These diaphoretic herbs have constituents that, when eaten, increase the blood circulation to the skin, which causes perspiration and ultimately lowers the fever.

GINGER WARMING TEA

10–12 thin slices of fresh ginger root
4 cups of water
Juice from 1 orange
Juice of ½ lemon
½ cup honey or maple syrup (optional)

Place ginger root and water in a pan and boil gently for 10 minutes. Strain. Add orange juice, lemon juice, and honey. Consume as a warming tea. Several large cups consumed in a row or drunk in a hot bath can elevate the body temperature and promote perspiration. This may help break a fever or reduce congestion.

Diaphoretic herbs include boneset, catnip, cinnamon, ginger, mint, thyme, and garlic. It is essential to drink plenty of fluids when taking these herbs, however, or dehydration may result. They're most effective when taken as hot teas. After drinking the tea, go to bed, wrap up in warm blankets, and sweat it out. Continue to drink plenty of fluids.

HEADACHE

The pain of a headache can be steady, piercing, or throbbing; its severity can range from minor discomfort to debilitation. Tension headaches and migraines are the most common types. Stress, irregular sleep, hormonal shifts, depression, and eyestrain, among other things, can trigger a headache.

Think away your pain. Yes, you can use your mind to heal your head. With biofeedback training, you can learn to control certain involuntary bodily functions, such as heart rate and body temperature, which can contribute to headaches. Take relaxation lessons from a biofeedback trainer and then practice at home. Wear loose clothing and sit in a comfortable chair. Close your eyes and imagine you are progressively tightening and releasing all your muscles, from your toes to the crown of your head.

Poke holes in it. Acupuncture has a good reputation for curing headaches, especially chronic ones like migraines. By inserting needles at specific points on the body, the acupuncturist promises to restore the flow of qi, the vital life force, throughout the body. Now able to heal itself, the body weathers the stressors that might otherwise cause headaches.

Pinch yourself. If needles aren't for you, you can gain benefits similar to those offered through acupuncture by practicing acupressure. For a headache, squeeze the energy point known as L14, on the web between the thumb and index finger.

You'll also find relief by massaging GB20, located on the back of the head at the base of the skull.

Get your neck straight. Even through it's your head that's hurting, a chiropractor is likely to relieve the pain by manipulating vertebrae in the neck.

Sit lotus-style. If you regularly practice the postures and breathing of yoga, you'll have fewer headaches, and the ones you get will be less severe.

Root for rosemary. Herbs containing rosmarinic acid act as anti-inflammatory agents, just like aspirin, ibuprofen, and acetaminophen do. These headache-busting herbs include rosemary and sage. Crush a handful of herbs and rub them on your temples or head. Or brew up herbal teas or add the plants to your bathwater.

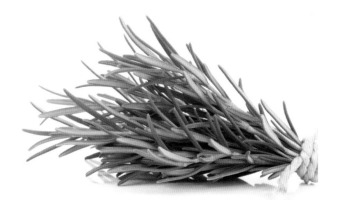

ROSEMARY AND SAGE TEA

A blended tea of rosemary and sage has also been used as a traditional folk remedy. Put one teaspoon of crushed rosemary leaves and one teaspoon of crushed sage leaves in a cup and fill with boiling water. Cover well to prevent the helpful substances from escaping. Let steep until the tea reaches room temperature. Drink ½ cup two to three times a day for two or three days.

Be a sourpuss. Soak a cloth in full strength vinegar, wring it out, gently apply it to the forehead, and lie down for 15 minutes to soothe headache pain.

Reach for the feverfew. Feverfew is used to relieve headaches, especially migraines, since it relaxes the blood vessels. Feverfew freeze-dried capsules and tablets are available are health stores. With fresh feverfew, you can also prepare a tea by using about 1 tablespoon of dried leaves per cup of hot water; steep for 10 minutes. Because feverfew does relax blood vessels, it can increase blood flow during menstruation. Because it can cause contractions, it should not be taken during pregnancy. Children should not take feverfew.

Use a cold compress. Cover your eyes with a washcloth dipped in ice-cold water or place an ice pack on the pain site. For many people, using ice as soon as possible after the onset of the headache will relieve the pain within 20 minutes.

Try heat. If you're cold to the idea of ice, try putting a warm washcloth over your eyes or on the site of the pain. Leave the compress on for half an hour, re-warming it as necessary.

Help from the kitchen. Peppermint and spearmint have been used as natural headache remedies because of their anti-inflammatory properties. Put one ounce of dried mint leaves in a one-quart jar and fill with boiling water. Cover tightly to prevent the escape of the aromatic constituents. Drink ½ cup of the tea two to four times a day.

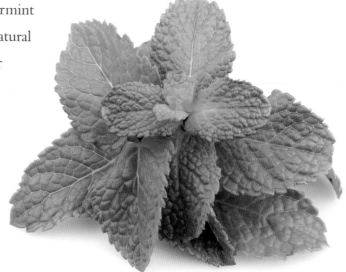

An apple a day. Inhaling the scent of apples may help soothe a migraine. You can get the benefit by cooking with apples, or you can use a high-quality apple-scented candle or air spray.

PAIN RELIEF

Pain is a sign that your body has been harmed by disease, injury, or abnormal changes. Pain can range from mild irritation to excruciating agony. Pain is among the most commonly reported symptoms and is linked to innumerable disorders and diseases. It can be acute, such as after an injury, or chronic, as with arthritis. Here are some ideas for how to counter the pain.

You can with cayenne. It's hard to believe that a substance that causes discomfort can help to relieve pain. Bite into a cayenne pepper and you'll imagine that your tongue is on fire. But apply cayenne externally, in the form of a lotion, ointment, salve, or liniment, and it will help relieve many kinds of pain.

Continue the herbal tradition. Many herbs have long been used to relieve pain, although we don't always know why they do so. These include cramp bark, willow bark, ginger, rosemary, angelica, and meadowsweet.

Breathe deeply. Smelling certain essential oils can help to ease muscles aches, spasms, and inflammation. Oils to try include ginger, marjoram, peppermint, and thyme.

Try a hands-on approach. It's natural to rub a spot that we've just bumped or massage an overworked muscle. But there may be more to it than simply instinct. Massage can help muscles to expect toxic chemicals. Many bodywork therapies can ease muscle pain and restore muscle function. Massage is particularly recommended to relieve muscle pain and tension.

Press the point. Reflexology applies pressure to certain reflex points on the feet and hands to help the body heal itself. Shiatsu involves finger therapy at certain points on the body, often places nowhere near the site of discomfort, to ease pain and improve circulation.

Flip a mental switch. There is no "switch" in our brains controlling painful sensation. But if you imagine that there is, and then mentally turn the switch off, you may attain some relief. Biofeedback training can be useful for muscle pain that refuses to go away. Biofeedback therapy teaches people to relax by tensing their muscles and then letting go. Patients can also learn to "switch off" pain signals in their brains.

Butter up. Tibetan doctors mix butter with herbs such as cardamom and sandalwood and apply the ointment to painful areas, such as the back. The herbs may also be powdered, burned, and inhaled to aid in healing pain.

Go for ginger. Ginger root powder may be useful in improving pain, stiffness, lack of mobility, and swelling. Larger dosages in the area of 3 or 4 grams of ginger powder daily appear most effective.

NERVE PAIN OIL

If pain is caused by a pinched nerve, try this aromatherapy recipe.

4 drops chamomile oil

3 drops marjoram oil

3 drops helichrysum oil (optional)

2 drops lavender oil

1 ounce vegetable oil

Combine all ingredients and store in a tightly capped jar. Apply as needed to relieve pain.

SKIN CONDITIONS & SUNBURN

Visible and uncomfortable, skin conditions demand attention. Perhaps that why there are so many traditional remedies for skin conditions, including acne, dry skin, eczema, and itching and rashes, such as those caused by poison ivy and poison oak. Almost everyone has suffered at one point or another from a sunburn, so this list contains some tips for that too—although if your sunburn is bad enough to cause blistering, seek help from your doctor.

Soak it away. For relief from eczema, throw a few handfuls of baking soda in a warm bath. The remedy is also used for relieving hives and other skin conditions. For sunburn, fill the tuba with lukewarm water, add a cup of baking soda, and soak for thirty to sixty minutes. When you're done, let your skin dry naturally. Don't chafe it with a towel.

Try a traditional poultice for acne. In China, folk healers treat acne by grinding dried mung beans, mixing the powder with water, and applying the poultice to the face, like a mask.

Reach for vinegar for poison ivy relief. A traditional remedy in Appalachia is to "wash away" poison ivy with vinegar. Vinegar works well to relieve any type of itching, including that caused by allergic rashes.

Pour yourself a cup of coffee... when you're suffering from poison ivy. Then pour it on yourself. Washing itchy skin with a strong cup of coffee (cooled, of course) has helped some people find relief from poison ivy.

Replace soap with...oatmeal? Next time your hands are chapped, try washing them with water and oatmeal. After drying your hands with a towel, rub them again with dry oatmeal.

Reduce puffiness with potatoes. Try a potato poultice to remove bags under your eyes. Clean and grate three unpeeled potatoes and press them with your hands to form a paste. Apply for fifteen minutes. Remove the paste and wash and dry the skin thoroughly.

Get milk. In the Southwest and in Appalachia, folk healers use milk and buttermilk to relieve skin irritation and discomfort.

Say hello to aloe. A widespread remedy in many cultures for minor burns and sunburn is to use the aloe plant's soothing sap. Slice the leaf down the middle and rub the goo on your skin. Or make a lotion by adding two ounces of fresh aloe vera sap to eight ounces of extra virgin olive oil.

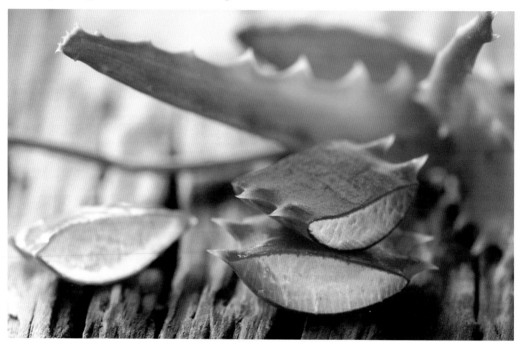

Get comfort from comfrey. Apply cold grated comfrey root or a cloth soaked in cool comfrey tea to sunburns or other minor burns. (Note that comfrey should not be used internally, only topically.)

Solve sunburn with vinegar. A mixture of white or apple cider vinegar with an equal amount of cool water can be used to bathe a garden-variety sunburn. If no one is around to help you, fill a spray bottle with the solution and spray the affected areas. You can also wear a large, loose-fitting, soft cotton T-shirt that has been soaked in the mixture.

STOMACH PROBLEMS

Ancient healers of Greece, India, and China believed that the digestive tract was the root of the tree of good health. With a healthy digestive tract, the body could readily absorb muscle- and bone-building nutrients from foods. Irregular or improperly functioning digestion can, indeed, cause or contribute to disease anywhere in the body. If you're experiencing nausea, pain in the stomach, or constipation, here are some things that may help.

Take your mother's advice. When you were little, your mother may have given you a glass of ginger ale when your tummy was upset. It's a remedy favored by moms around the world, from New England to Saudi Arabia to the Caribbean. Ginger does help settle your stomach—Mom knows best!

Note that to be effective, you should be drinking real ginger ale, not just ginger-flavored soda. Or you can make ginger tea. Stir half a teaspoon of ground ginger into one cup of hot water and steep for about five minutes. Drink up to three cups a day.

Avail yourself of an Arabian remedy. Chew caraway seeds to relieve gas and ease digestion. It's a remedy that's been used for centuries in cultures around the world, particularly in the Middle East. In fact, in India and the Middle East, thoughtful hosts pass a small bowl of caraway or fennel seeds for guests to nibble after sumptuous meals.

Keep it topical. Apply a hot compress to the abdomen after heavy meals. Presumably, the heat attracts circulation to the area, thus improving digestion, although the remedy may first have been used simply because it feels soothing.

Use your nose. Merely inhaling the scent of certain essential oils, according to aromatherapists, can improve digestion and eliminate gas. Useful digestive herb oils include black pepper *(Piper nigrum)*, clary sage, juniper berry, lemongrass, peppermint, rosemary, and thyme.

Open sesame. Sesame seeds have been used as a folk remedy for constipation. They're nutritious and contain lots of oil, which helps to moisten the intestines. Adding ½ ounce of sesame seeds a day to your diet may help; you can sprinkle ground seeds on foods like a condiment.

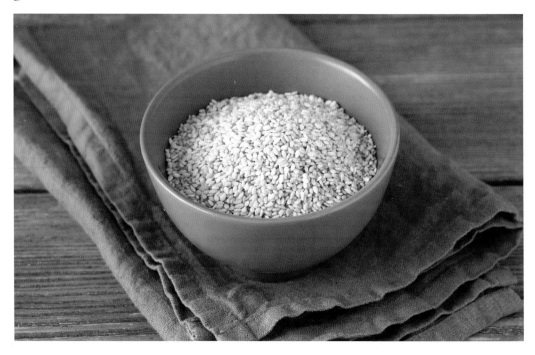

Spice up your life. A variety of plants appear to work on the digestive system. You can try anise, basil, caraway, coriander, and fennel to stimulate digestion. Rosemary is said to improve food absorption and peppermint treats irritable bowel syndrome. Basil can help overcome nausea, even nausea from chemotherapy. Lemongrass is used in Brazil, the Caribbean, and Southeast Asia to relieve nervous stomachs.

Go for the grape. To relieve constipation, one traditional remedy is an herb called the Oregon grape. The root of this plant and some close cousins such as barberry have been used safely since ancient times to overcome occasional constipation. Mix ½ teaspoon Oregon grape tincture in water and sip slowly before eating for best results.

Apple it up. To relieve heartburn, munch on a fresh, unpeeled (but thoroughly washed) apple.

Add in vinegar. To ease nausea, such as the nausea of morning sickness, stir 1 teaspoon apple cider vinegar into a glass of water and drink it.

CHAMOMILE TEA RECIPE

This all-purpose tea is useful for nausea, irritable bowel, ulcers, and colitis. Omit the licorice is you have high blood pressure.

German chamomile flowers
Licorice root, shredded
Fennel seeds
Peppermint

Combine equal parts of dry herbs and steep 1 tablespoon of the mixture in a cup of hot water for 15 minutes. Strain and drink 2 or more cups a day as needed for gastrointestinal issues.

TUMMY OIL

2 drops lemongrass oil

1 drop fennel oil

2 drops chamomile oil

2 ounces vegetable oil

Combine the ingredients and massage all over the abdominal area. This all-purpose aromatherapy formula will thwart indigestion, including nausea, gas, appetite loss, and motion sickness, as well as help improve appetite and digestion. You can also add 1 to 2 teaspoons to bathwater. Use as needed. Feel free to alter this formula by choosing other oils that aid digestion such as clary sage, rosemary, and basil. Be careful of hot oils like thyme, peppermint, and black pepper, especially in a bath since they can burn the skin.